1200
Multiple Choice
Questions in
Pharmacology

1200 Multiple Choice Questions in Pharmacology

R.W. Foster (Editor), J.R. Carpenter, B. Cox, M.J. Dascombe,
M. Hollingsworth, N.P. Keaney, G.E. Mawer, I.D. Morris,
P.W. Mullen, J.M.H. Rees, H. Schneiden, A.P. Silverman,
R.C. Small, Janet Vale, A.H. Weston, E.T. Whalley, T.R. Wilson

Staff of the Department of Pharmacology,
Materia Medica and Therapeutics, The University of Manchester

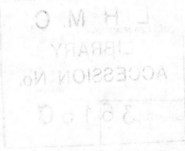
BUTTERWORTHS
LONDON · BOSTON
Sydney · Wellington · Durban · Toronto

United Kingdom London	Butterworth & Co (Publishers) Ltd 88 Kingsway, WC2B 6AB
Australia Sydney	Butterworth Pty Ltd 586 Pacific Highway, Chatswood, NSW 2067 Also at Melbourne, Brisbane, Adelaide and Perth
Canada Toronto	Butterworth & Co (Canada) Ltd 2265 Midland Avenue, Scarborough, Ontario, M1P 4S1
New Zealand Wellington	Butterworths of New Zealand Ltd T & W Young Building, 77–85 Customhouse Quay, 1, CPO Box 472
South Africa Durban	Butterworth & Co (South Africa) Ltd 152–154 Gale Street
USA Boston	Butterworth (Publishers) Inc 10 Tower Office Park, Woburn, Mass. 01801

First published 1980

© University of Manchester, Department of Pharmacology, Materia Medica and Therapeutics 1980

ISBN 0 407 00192 1

British Library Cataloguing in Publication Data

1200 multiple choice questions in pharmacology.
1. Pharmacology – Problems, exercises, etc.
I. Foster, R W II. Twelve hundred multiple
choice questions in pharmacology
615'.1'076   RM105   79-42816

ISBN 0-407-00192-1

Typeset in England by Scribe Design, Gillingham, Kent.
Printed and bound in America

Preface

This selection of multiple choice questions in pharmacology is offered in the hope that it may be found useful in any of four different ways:

1 As a source of ready-made questions for use by examiners
2 As a source of ideas which may aid examiners in the construction of new questions
3 As an aid to candidates in practising multiple choice examination technique
4 As a means by which students can assess their own progress in acquiring pharmacological knowledge

The questions have been designed, debated, amended, tested and revised over the last 6 years. They have been used in the assessment of students of medicine and pharmacy and other groups of science students reading pharmacology as either a main or subsidiary subject. The large majority have also had the benefit of scrutiny by external examiners.

Some of the questions test mental functions other than factual recall but it is freely admitted that most are at the simpler level. It has become fashionable to berate questions which 'merely' test factual knowledge but we repudiate such a view when applied to the assessment of students early in their academic experience of a subject. Higher objectives require a bedrock of fact before they can be exercised.

The questions are classified only in the broadest way by subject matter into seven themes. Within each theme they are classified on structural grounds into the types expounded below, although not all types of questions have been used in every theme. The time required to read, think about and answer one question is very variable but over any reasonably sized sample of questions an average allowance of one minute for each has been found generous by our students.

The answers appear at the back and, where available, a figure is provided showing the facility of the question. This is derived from the average proportion of candidates correctly answering the question over all the occasions when it has been used in formal examinations. It is our experience that these figures are reasonably reproducible and have predictive value. It is likely that the precise numbers will only be locally relevant but they are offered in the hope that the relative sizes will be helpful.

Policy on drug names

We have used the names approved by the British Pharmacopoeia Commission and excluded trade names save in the very rare instances where no approved name has been assigned. For readers who are more familiar with North American terminology the US Pharmacopeia name has been included in square brackets in the text after every occurrence of the name. Only significant differences, however, have been declared; we have not bothered to draw special attention to systematic differences arising from different spelling conventions such as -ph- (-f-) and -oe- (-e-). Neither did -trophin (-tropin) nor -barbitone (-barbital) seem likely to mystify our readers.

Acknowledgements

We thank Roger C. Small for preparing the diagrams, Beryl A. Foster for typing the manuscript and Michael Hollingsworth, Niall P. Keaney, George E. Mawer, Ian D. Morris, John M.H. Rees, Roger C. Small and Janet Vale for proofreading sections of the typescript.

The Types of Questions and their General Rubrics

Type 1 (one correct from n)

The reader must choose for each question the one correct answer or completion from a list of up to nine answer or completion options.
General rubric: Select the one most suitable response from the options provided.

Type 2 (one correct from n but a group of two or more questions has the same rubric and set of options)

The reader must choose for each question the one correct answer or completion from a list of up to nine answer or completion options.
General rubric: For each question in the following group select the one most suitable response from the options provided. Each option may be used more than once.

Type 3 (single precoded set from n)

The reader must choose the letter corresponding to the appropriate combination of options since each individual option may be either appropriate or inappropriate.
General rubric: None — a specific rubric is supplied.

Type 4 (matched pairs)

The reader must match an option to each question; the number of options is equal to or greater than the number of questions, subject to a limit of nine options.

General rubric: In the following group of questions match the most appropriate option with each question number. No option may be used more than once.

Type 5 (passage completion)

The reader must fill each gap in a passage by choosing the one correct completion from a list of up to nine completion options.

General rubric: In the following passage words or phrases have been omitted and replaced by key numbers. Select the one most suitable word or phrase from the appropriate list of options to fill each gap. Note that a key may appear more than once; the option selected must be appropriate for all occurrences.

Type 6 (quantitative comparison)

The reader must compare in a quantitative sense the two entities described in a pair of statements.

General rubric: Each question consists of two statements, X and Y. Compare X and Y quantitatively and select:

A if X is greater than Y
B if X and Y are approximately equal
C if Y is greater than X

Type 7 (causal quantitative relationship)

The reader must decide whether, and in which direction, a change in one entity causes a change in a second.

General rubric: Each question consists of two entities, X and Y. Select:

A if change in X leads to change in Y in the same direction
B if change in X does not lead to change in Y
C if change in X leads to change in Y in the opposite direction

Type 8 (causal relationship)

The reader must establish not only whether each statement of a pair is true or false but also whether there is a causal relationship between the two. Each question consists of an assertion and a reason. Select:

A if the assertion and reason are true statements and the reason is the correct explanation of the assertion
B if the assertion and reason are true statements but the reason is *not* a correct explanation of the assertion
C if the assertion is true but the reason is a false statement
D if the assertion is false but the reason is a true statement
E if both assertion and reason are ~~true~~ statements
   false.

Type 9 (one incorrect from *n*)

The reader must choose the one incorrect answer or completion from a list of up to nine answer or completion options.
General rubric: Select the **ONE INCORRECT** response from the options provided.

Contents

1 Autonomic Pharmacology

including skeletal muscle, local anaesthetics
and anti-arrhythmics

Type 1

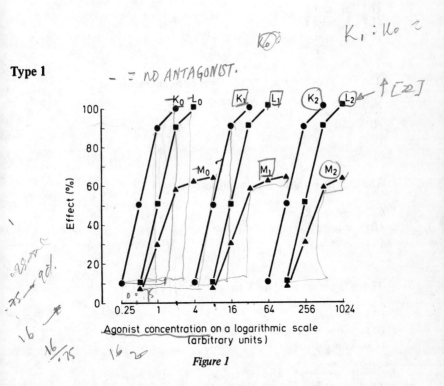

Figure 1

Figure 1 presents a family of curves of agonist concentration against effect.
Curves K_0, L_0, M_0 were obtained for three different agonists in the absence
of any antagonist. Curves K_1, L_1, M_1 were obtained for the same three
agonists in the presence of a low concentration of antagonist X. Curves K_2,
L_2, M_2 were obtained for the same three agonists in the presence of a higher
concentration of the antagonist X.
Use Figure 1 for questions 1–6.

1   The agonists K and L act upon:

    (A)   different receptor sites

    (B)   the same receptor site and this is identical to the receptor site for agonist M

    (C)   the same receptor site but this is different from the receptor site for agonist M

2   The most potent agonist is:

    (A)   agonist K

    (B)   agonist L

    (C)   agonist M

3   The ED_{90} for agonist L in the absence of antagonist is:

    (A)   0.5

    (B)   2.0

    (C)   16

4   The agonist with the smallest efficacy is:

    (A)   agonist K

    (B)   agonist L

    (C)   agonist M

5   The antagonism of M by X is:

    (A)   irreversible

    (B)   non-competitive

    (C)   competitive

6   The ratio, potency of agonist K in the presence of the lower concentration of X : potency of agonist K in the absence of X is:

    (A)   1 : 2

    (B)   2 : 1

    (C)   1 : 4

    (D)   4 : 1

(E)   1 : 8
(F)   8 : 1
(G)   1 : 16
(H)   16 : 1

A drug, D, combines with a receptor, R, to form a drug-receptor complex DR. The reaction obeys the law of Mass Action and may be expressed by the following equation:

$$D + R \underset{k_2}{\overset{k_1}{\rightleftharpoons}} DR$$

Let   [D] = molar concentration of free drug
      [R] = molar concentration of free (unoccupied) receptor
      [DR] = molar concentration of drug-receptor complex

The association rate constant for the reaction, k_1, has the value $10 \, \ell \, mol^{-1} \, s^{-1}$.

The dissociation rate constant for the reaction, k_2, has the value $0.001 \, s^{-1}$.

Use this information for questions 7–10.

7   The equilibrium affinity constant, K_a, is given by the expression:

(A) $k_2 \times [DR]/(k_1 \times [D] \times [R])$
(B) $k_1 \times [D] \times [R]/(k_2 \times [DR])$
(C) $[DR]/([D] \times [R])$
(D) $[D] \times [R]/[DR]$

8   The units of K_a will be:

(A) $\ell \, mol^{-1}$
(B) $mol \, \ell^{-1}$
(C) s^{-1}
(D) $s \, mol^{-1}$

9   For occupancy of 50% of receptors at equilibrium the molar concentration of free drug will be:

(A)   0.1
(B)   0.01
(C)   0.001
(D)   0.0001

10   Assume that the observed response is proportional to the fraction of
      receptors occupied (Clark's occupation hypothesis). What will the
      observed response (as a percentage of maximum) be when the equili-
      brium concentration of free drug is 0.001 M?

      (A)   0.091%
      (B)   0.91%
      (C)   9.1%
      (D)   91%

11   A new drug, tested in man by intravenous injection, causes mild tachy-
      cardia but no change in mean arterial blood pressure. The drug causes
      dilation of the pupil and reduces the activity of the eccrine sweat
      glands, but does not interfere with ejaculation. Given that the drug
      does not penetrate the blood/brain barrier, the drug is most likely to
      act as:

      (A)   an agonist at α-adrenoceptors
      (B)   an antagonist at α-adrenoceptors
      (C)   an agonist at β-adrenoceptors
      (D)   an antagonist at β-adrenoceptors
      (E)   an agonist at muscarinic cholinoceptors
      (F)   an antagonist at muscarinic cholinoceptors
      (G)   an agonist at the nicotinic cholinoceptors of ganglia
      (H)   an antagonist at the nicotinic cholinoceptors of ganglia

12   A new drug, tested in man by intramuscular injection, lowers the mean
      arterial blood pressure, causes diarrhoea and mild pupillary constric-
      tion, but does not influence salivary secretion. Given that the drug does
      not penetrate the blood/brain barrier, its most likely mechanism of
      action is:

      (A)   the activation of muscarinic cholinoceptors
      (B)   the activation of α-adrenoceptors
      (C)   the activation of β-adrenoceptors
      (D)   the stimulation of baroreceptors
      (E)   blockade of transmission through autonomic ganglia
      (F)   inhibition of the release of transmitter from postganglionic para-
            sympathetic nerve terminals
      (G)   inhibition of the release of transmitter from postganglionic sym-
            pathetic nerve terminals

13 The drug whose molecular structure is indicated above:

(A) is an indirectly acting sympathomimetic

(B) is less potent than isoprenaline [isoproterenol] in evoking contraction of vascular smooth muscle

(C) is less potent than methoxamine in evoking contraction of vascular smooth muscle

(D) is metabolised by catechol-*O*-methyltransferase and/or monoamine oxidase

(E) is most effective in stimulating the heart when in the form of its dextrorotatory isomer

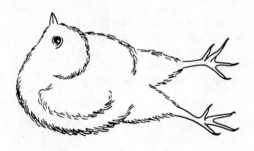

Figure 2

14 Which drug, when administered to a chick by intravenous injection, would have produced blockade of neuromuscular transmission with the features indicated in *Figure 2*?

(A) botulinus toxin

(B) hemicholinium

(C) pancuronium

(D) suxamethonium [succinylcholine]

(E) tetrodotoxin

(F) none of the above drugs

, ↓ Ach receptors

A patient suffering from <u>myasthenia gravis</u> has been undergoing a course of treatment with neostigmine and atropine. He unexpectedly develops excessive muscular weakness. On injection of edrophonium the patient's condition is temporarily exacerbated.
Use this information for questions 15–17.   *few seconds action*

15   Treatment of the patient with neostigmine and atropine was:

    (A)   curative – corrects the defect which is the cause of the disease
    (B)   prophylactic – prevents the occurrence of subsequent attacks of the disease
    (C)   symptomatic – relieves the symptoms of the disease without correcting the underlying defect
    (D)   short term – may safely and permanently be discontinued after a few days

16   The exacerbation of the patient's condition induced by edrophonium suggests:

    (A)   he has received too little atropine
    (B)   he has received too much atropine
    (C)   he has received too little neostigmine
    (D)   he has received too much neostigmine
    (E)   his disease has increased in severity

17   The exacerbation of the patient's condition induced by edrophonium prompts the prescribing of:

    (A)   more atropine
    (B)   less atropine
    (C)   more neostigmine
    (D)   less neostigmine
    (E)   pancuronium

18   Procaine is eliminated from blood plasma mainly by:

    (A)   excretion unchanged in the urine
    (B)   oxidative metabolism in the liver
    (C)   redistribution into adipose tissue
    (D)   hydrolysis brought about by cholinesterase (pseudocholinesterase)

A piece of smooth muscle is richly innervated by noradrenergic neurones. The smooth muscle cells contain α-adrenoceptors (which mediate contraction) but not β-adrenoceptors. The effects of noradrenaline [norepinephrine], adrenaline [epinephrine], methoxamine and isoprenaline [isoproterenol] upon this tissue are examined both prior to, and after, the administration of a concentration of cocaine which inhibits the neuronal uptake of noradrenaline [norepinephrine].
Use this information for questions 19–21.

19 Treatment of the tissue with cocaine:

(A) decreases the potency of noradrenaline [norepinephrine] relative to isoprenaline [isoproterenol]

(B) increases the potency of noradrenaline [norepinephrine] relative to isoprenaline [isoproterenol]

(C) does not change the potency of noradrenaline [norepinephrine] relative to isoprenaline [isoproterenol]

20 Treatment of the tissue with cocaine:

(A) decreases the potency of methoxamine relative to isoprenaline [isoproterenol]

(B) increases the potency of methoxamine relative to isoprenaline [isoproterenol]

(C) does not change the potency of methoxamine relative to isoprenaline [isoproterenol]

21 After treatment of the tissue with cocaine the expected relative order of agonist potency is:

(A) methoxamine > noradrenaline [norepinephrine] ≏ adrenaline [epinephrine] > isoprenaline [isoproterenol]

(B) isoprenaline [isoproterenol] > noradrenaline [norepinephrine] ≏ adrenaline [epinephrine] > methoxamine

(C) noradrenaline [norepinephrine] ≏ adrenaline [epinephrine] > methoxamine > isoprenaline [isoproterenol]

(D) methoxamine > isoprenaline [isoproterenol] > noradrenaline [norepinephrine] ≏ adrenaline [epinephrine]

22   Concentrations of an anticholinesterase drug, X, which inhibit acetyl-cholinesterase activity in tissue homogenates, produce a similar inhibition of the cholinesterase (pseudocholinesterase) activity of serum. The inhibitory activity of X markedly increases when the pH of the medium is changed from 10 to 6. Homogenates whose esterase activity has been inhibited by X can be reactivated by dialysis. Drug X is likely to be:

(A)   ecothiopate [echothiophate]
(B)   dyflos
(C)   malathion
(D)   neostigmine
(E)   physostigmine (eserine)

23   Suxamethonium [succinylcholine] has produced prolonged muscle paralysis in a patient. It is deduced that:

(A)   the patient has poor renal function
(B)   he has suffered prolonged competitive neuromuscular blockade
(C)   his plasma cholinesterase activity is low or atypical
(D)   the suxamethonium [succinylcholine] has been mixed with sodium thiopentone with which it is incompatible
(E)   suxamethonium [succinylcholine] cannot be accurately standardised, and an overdose has thus been given

24   The muscarinic receptor blocking agent hyoscine [scopolamine] hydrobromide (0.4 mg) may be preferred to atropine sulphate (0.6 mg) for pre-operative medication because it has:

(A)   shorter duration of action on bronchial glands
(B)   greater duration of action on bronchial glands
(C)   less intense action on bronchial glands
(D)   more intense action on bronchial glands
(E)   less sedative effect
(F)   greater sedative effect

25   Lignocaine [lidocaine] and propranolol are both:

(A)   antagonists at β-adrenoceptors
(B)   used to correct cardiac arrhythmias
(C)   liable to induce bronchospasm
(D)   contraindicated in patients with hypertension

26 Both bethanidine and pentolinium:

(A) cause adrenergic neurone blockade
(B) cause autonomic ganglion blockade
(C) cause orthostatic hypotension
(D) are well absorbed from the gastrointestinal tract

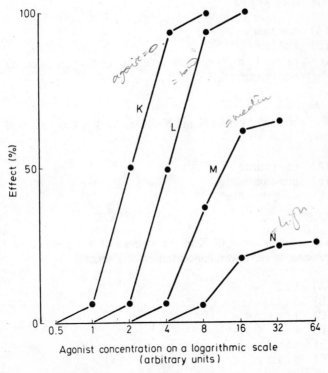

Figure 3

Figure 3 represents a family of curves of concentration against effect for an agonist drug X. Curve K was the control curve obtained in the absence of any agonist. Curve L was obtained in the presence of a low concentration of antagonist Y. Curve M was obtained in the presence of a medium concentration of antagonist Y. Curve N was obtained in the presence of a high concentration of antagonist Y.
Use this information for questions 27–32.

27   The ED_{50} for X in the absence of Y was.

(A)   0.5
(B)   1.0
(C)   1.5
(D)   2.0
(E)   3.0

28   The efficacy of X:

(A)   was high
(B)   was low
(C)   cannot be assigned a low or high value since insufficient data have
      been presented

29   Examination of curves M and N shows that the antagonism of X by Y
      was:

(A)   competitive
(B)   non-competitive
(C)   surmountable

30   The ratio, potency of X in the absence of Y : potency of X in the
      presence of the lowest concentration of Y was:

(A)   1 : 2
(B)   2 : 1
(C)   1 : 4
(D)   4 : 1
(E)   1.5 : 4
(F)   4 : 1.5

31   In order to elicit a maximal response in the absence of antagonist, the
      fraction of receptors requiring activation:

(A)   was 100%
(B)   was less than 100%
(C)   cannot be assigned a value equal to or less than 100% since insuf-
      ficient data have been presented

32   Antagonism of the type illustrated by *Figure 3* occurs between:

(A)   phentolamine and noradrenaline [norepinephrine] acting on arterial smooth muscle

(B)   propranolol and noradrenaline [norepinephrine] acting on bronchiolar smooth muscle

(C)   phenoxybenzamine and noradrenaline [norepinephrine] acting on arterial smooth muscle

A new sympathomimetic drug (a catecholamine) was tested for activity on various tissues isolated from the cat. Values for the ED_{50} of the new drug were:

1×10^{-5} M for increasing the force of cardiac contraction
1×10^{-7} M for contraction of arterial smooth muscle
5×10^{-4} M for relaxation of bronchiolar smooth muscle
2×10^{-7} M for contraction of the nictitating membrane

These ED_{50} values were not changed by pretreatment of the tissues with cocaine or by pretreatment of the animals with reserpine.
Use this information for questions 33–35.

33   The new drug is likely to be:

(A)   an indirectly acting sympathomimetic

(B)   a directly acting sympathomimetic which selectively activates β-adrenoceptors

(C)   a directly acting sympathomimetic which selectively activates α-adrenoceptors

(D)   a directly acting sympathomimetic which does not selectively activate either α- or β-adrenoceptors

34   When given by intravenous infusion to an anaesthetised cat at a rate sufficient to raise the systolic blood pressure by 20 mmHg, the drug is likely to:

(A)   lower markedly the diastolic blood pressure and increase the heart rate

(B)   have no significant effect on diastolic blood pressure or heart rate

(C)   raise the diastolic blood pressure and increase the heart rate

(D)   raise the diastolic blood pressure and decrease the heart rate

35   The cardiovascular effects of the new drug *in vivo* are likely to be terminated principally by:

   (A)   excretion of the unchanged drug in the urine
   (B)   biotransformation to inactive metabolites
   (C)   uptake of the drug into noradrenergic neurones

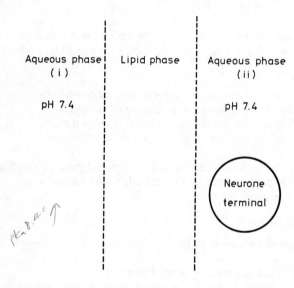

Figure 4

In *Figure 4* a lipid barrier separates two aqueous phases each with a pH of 7.4. A local anaesthetic with a pK_a of 8.4 is dissolved in aqueous phase (i). A neurone terminal devoid of any sheath is present in aqueous phase (ii). You are given that $pK_a = pH - \log_{10}$ ([unionised base]/[cation])
Use this information for questions 36–40.

36   What proportion of the drug in aqueous phase (i) exists as the unionised base:

   (A)   0.9%
   (B)   9.0%
   (C)   90%
   (D)   99%

37   Raising the pH of aqueous phase (i) would:

   (A)   facilitate entry of the drug into the lipid phase
   (B)   reduce the entry of the drug into the lipid phase
   (C)   have no effect on the entry of the drug into the lipid phase

38   Following the penetration of the drug into aqueous phase (ii) raising the pH of that phase would:

   (A)   facilitate the anaesthetic action of the drug on the neurone terminal
   (B)   reduce the anaesthetic action of the drug on the neurone terminal
   (C)   have no effect upon the anaesthetic action of the drug on the neurone terminal

39   Following penetration of the drug into aqueous phase (ii) raising the Ca^{2+} concentration of that phase would:

   (A)   facilitate the anaesthetic action of the drug upon the neurone
   (B)   reduce the anaesthetic action of the drug upon the neurone
   (C)   have no effect on the anaesthetic action of the drug on the neurone

40   Following the penetration of the drug into aqueous phase (ii) raising the concentration of Na^+ in that phase would:

   (A)   facilitate the anaesthetic action of the drug on the neurone
   (B)   reduce the anaesthetic action of the drug on the neurone
   (C)   have no effect on the anaesthetic action of the drug on the neurone

Type 2

Which chemical transmitter is released from the axon terminals and what effect has this transmitter on the postsynaptic cell?

41   A postganglionic neurone supplying the ciliary muscle
42   A neurone supplying adrenal medullary chromaffin cells

43   A postganglionic neurone arising from a synapse within the heart tissue and supplying the sinoatrial node
44   A postganglionic neurone supplying the dilator pupillae
45   A postganglionic neurone of a pathway arising from the thoracic region of the spinal cord and supplying the smooth muscle of the spleen
46   A neurone supplying the ventricular myocardium

Options for 41–46:

    (A)   acetylcholine released; excitatory effect
    (B)   acetylcholine released; inhibitory effect
    (C)   noradrenaline [norepinephrine] released; excitatory effect
    (D)   noradrenaline [norepinephrine] released; inhibitory effect

47   Ether has an effect at the skeletal neuromuscular junction which resembles that of:
48   Poisoning by organophosphorus anticholinesterases, if detected early, can be effectively treated with:
49   The action of tubocurarine at the skeletal neuromuscular junction can be antagonised by:

Options for 47–49:

    (A)   pancuronium
    (B)   pentolinium
    (C)   pralidoxime
    (D)   pyridostigmine

With which site(s) in the active centre of cholinesterase does each of the drugs associate?

50   edrophonium
51   dyflos
52   acetylcholine
53   pyridostigmine

Options for 50–53:

    (A)   the anionic site only
    (B)   the esteratic site only
    (C)   both the anionic and esteratic sites

Which enzyme best answers the following descriptions?

54   Facilitates an esterification reaction which is the final stage in the synthesis of a neurotransmitter

55   Of the enzymes which hydrolyse acetylcholine, this is the more susceptible to inhibition by organophosphorus derivatives

56   Plays a minor role in terminating the effects of neurally released noradrenaline [norepinephrine] by converting it to methylated metabolites

57   After inhibition of this enzyme a patient must be warned not to eat tyramine-containing foodstuffs

58   Facilitates the rate-limiting step in the biosynthesis of noradrenaline [norepinephrine]

Options for 54–58:

(A)   acetylcholinesterase
(B)   catechol-*O*-methyltransferase (COMT)
(C)   choline acetyltransferase (cholineacetylase)
(D)   cholinesterase (pseudocholinesterase)
(E)   DOPA decarboxylase
(F)   dopamine-β-oxidase
(G)   monoamine oxidase (MAO)
(H)   phenylethanolamine-*N*-methyltransferase
(I)   tyrosine hydroxylase

Which drug best answers each description?

59   A drug which antagonises the effect of acetylcholine and that of splanchnic nerve stimulation on the chromaffin cells of the adrenal medulla

60   A drug which antagonises the effects of motor nerve stimulation on an end-plate of a skeletal muscle cell but not that of iontophoretically applied acetylcholine

61   A drug which antagonises the vasoconstrictor effect of both noradrenaline [norepinephrine] and tyramine

62   A drug which antagonises the vasoconstrictor effect of tyramine but not that of noradrenaline [norepinephrine]

63   A drug which antagonises the effects of both noradrenaline [norepinephrine] and tyramine on bronchiolar smooth muscle

Options for 59–63:

(A)   atropine
(B)   botulinus toxin

    (C)   guanethidine
    (D)   pentolinium
    (E)   phentolamine
    (F)   propranolol
    (G)   tubocurarine

A group of animals has been pretreated with reserpine. How would each of the responses be influenced by this pretreatment?

64   The change in heart rate caused by isoprenaline [isoproterenol]
65   The change in pupil diameter caused by ephedrine eyedrops
66   The immediate fall in blood pressure which occurs on tilting from the horizontal to the vertical (head up) position
67   The change in pupil diameter caused by cocaine eyedrops

Options for 64–67:

    (A)   pretreatment increases response
    (B)   pretreatment does not consistently affect the response
    (C)   pretreatment reduces response
    (D)   pretreatment reverses the response

Which drug pretreatment enhances the following pharmacological responses?

68   The cardiovascular response to eating ripe Stilton cheese
69   The response of the sinoatrial node to efferent vagal nerve impulses
70   The response of the Purkinje fibres of the isolated heart to isoprenaline [isoproterenol]

Options for 68–70:

    (A)   none of B to E
    (B)   cocaine
    (C)   imipramine
    (D)   neostigmine
    (E)   phenelzine

Which substance best fits each description?

71   A drug which is metabolised to give a false transmitter
72   A pharmacologically inactive breakdown product of both noradrenaline [norepinephrine] and adrenaline [epinephrine]

73   A drug which selectively antagonises the effects of catecholamines on cardiac β-adrenoceptors

74   A drug that can dilate the bronchioles at a dose which has little effect on the heart

Options for 71–74:

(A)   α-methyldopa
(B)   bethanidine
(C)   ephedrine
(D)   3-methoxy-4-hydroxymandelic acid (VMA)
(E)   phenelzine
(F)   practolol
(G)   pyrogallol
(H)   reserpine
(I)   salbutamol

Which is the most potent blocking agent of transmission between neurone and effector cell?

75   A postganglionic neurone supplying the ciliary muscle

76   The postganglionic neurone of a pathway arising from the sacral region of the spinal cord and supplying the propulsive musculature of the colon

77   A postganglionic neurone supplying an eccrine sweat gland

78   A neurone supplying adrenal medullary chromaffin cells

79   A small motor neurone supplying frog slow skeletal muscle cells

80   A postganglionic neurone supplying a blood vessel of the external genital erectile tissue

81   A neurone arising from the superior cervical ganglion of the cat and supplying the nictitating membrane

82   A neurone arising from the superior cervical ganglion and supplying the iris

83   A postganglionic neurone supplying the vas deferens or seminal vesicle

84   A neurone supplying the ventricular myocardium

Options for 75–84:

(A)   atropine
(B)   pentolinium
(C)   phentolamine
(D)   propranolol
(E)   tubocurarine

Which region of the mammalian heart best fits each description?

85   The region whose cells have the fastest inherent rate of action potential firing

86   The region mediating the bradycardia induced by vagal nerve stimulation

87   The region in which acetylcholine and noradrenaline [norepinephrine] have qualitatively similar effects on the refractory period

88   The region in which the propagation of the cardiac excitation wave is slowest

89   The region in which the ameliorative effects of digoxin in the treatment of a patient with atrial fibrillation are mediated

90   The usual site of origin of the ventricular arrhythmias induced by toxic concentrations of digoxin

91   The region in which the ameliorative effects of digoxin are mediated in the treatment of congestive heart failure with sinus rhythm

Options for 85–91:

(A)   sinoatrial node
(B)   atrial myocardium
(C)   atrioventricular node
(D)   Purkinje fibres
(E)   ventricular myocardium

Which is the best description of the mechanism of action of each hypotensive drug?

92   bethanidine
93   glyceryltrinitrate
94   pentolinium
95   veratridine

Options for 92–95

(A)   stimulation of the afferent limb of a depressor reflex arc
(B)   blockade of impulse transmission in vasoconstrictor pathways at ganglia
(C)   replacement of the stored neurotransmitter in adrenergic nerve endings by a false transmitter
(D)   depletion of stored neurotransmitter from adrenergic nerve endings, without replacement by a false transmitter

(E) blockade of action potential transmission in adrenergic pathways by an action on postganglionic nerve terminals

(F) occupation of receptor sites on smooth muscle cells of blood vessels, thus excluding a vasoconstrictor transmitter

(G) occupation of receptor sites on cardiac cells, thus excluding a cardiac-stimulant transmitter

(H) direct dilator action on blood vessels

Which mechanism of inhibition best describes each drug interaction?

96 Adrenaline [epinephrine] reduces the bronchoconstrictor effect of histamine

97 Adrenaline [epinephrine] reduces the effect of histamine on capillary permeability

98 Aminophylline reduces the bronchoconstrictor effect of histamine

99 Atropine reduces the action of acetylcholine on heart rate

100 Propranolol reduces the effect of adrenaline [epinephrine] on cardiac excitability

101 Phenoxybenzamine reduces the vasoconstrictor effect of noradrenaline [norepinephrine]

102 Neostigmine reduces the rate of hydrolysis of acetylcholine by acetylcholinesterase

103 Phenelzine reduces the rate of deamination of tyramine by monoamine oxidase

104 Dyflos reduces the rate of hydrolysis of acetylcholine by cholinesterase

Options for 96–104:

(A) inhibition by neutralisation: the drug and inhibitor combine to produce an inactive product

(B) functional inhibition: the drug and inhibitor produce opposite effects by acting on independent sites

(C) competitive inhibition: the drug and inhibitor are in mass action equilibrium with the same site of action

(D) non-surmountable inhibition: the inhibitor cannot be displaced from its site of action by increasing drug concentration

Which drug best fits each of the following descriptions?

105 A drug which, in sublocal anaesthetic concentrations, potentiates the actions of noradrenaline [norepinephrine]

106   A local anaesthetic drug which has a potent anorexic (appetite suppressant) action
107   The local anaesthetic which contains an amide linkage in its molecule and is used intravenously to control cardiac arrhythmias
108   A local anaesthetic which is poorly soluble in water and is only used as a topical anaesthetic
109   A short-acting local anaesthetic which has a marked vasodilator action

Options for 106–109:

    (A)   cocaine
    (B)   procaine
    (C)   lignocaine [lidocaine]
    (D)   tetrodotoxin
    (E)   ethyl chloride
    (F)   benzocaine

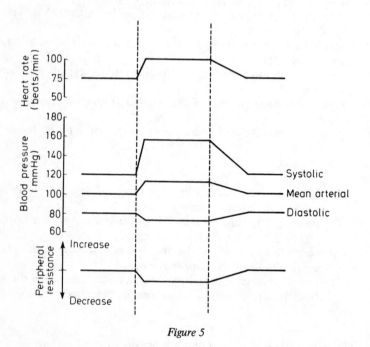

Figure 5

Figure 5 represents the cardiovascular effects seen in man during the intravenous infusion of adrenaline [epinephrine] (between the broken lines).
Use this information for questions 110–118.

110 Select the drug which, when given by intravenous infusion in man, shares the effect of adrenaline [epinephrine] upon the heart rate

111 Select the drug which, when given by intravenous infusion in man, produces the same effect as adrenaline [epinephrine] upon the peripheral resistance

Options for 110–111:

    (A)   methoxamine
    (B)   noradrenaline [norepinephrine]
    (C)   phenylephrine
    (D)   isoprenaline [isoproterenol]

112 These effects of intravenously infused adrenaline [epinephrine] upon the peripheral resistance in man are principally mediated by:

113 The effects of intravenously infused noradrenaline [norepinephrine] upon peripheral resistance in man are principally mediated by:

Options for 112–113:

    (A)   interaction of the drug with α-adrenoceptors of blood vessels
    (B)   interaction of the drug with β-adrenoceptors of the arterioles of skeletal muscle
    (C)   a reflex decrease in sympathetic discharge to the blood vessels resulting from the change in mean arterial blood pressure
    (D)   a reflex increase in sympathetic discharge to the blood vessels resulting from the change in mean arterial blood pressure

114 Intravenous infusion of noradrenaline [norepinephrine] in man has qualitatively similar effects to intravenous infusion of adrenaline [epinephrine] upon:

    (A)   pulse rate
    (B)   systolic blood pressure
    (C)   diastolic blood pressure
    (D)   peripheral resistance

115 These effects of adrenaline [epinephrine] upon the heart rate are principally mediated by:

116 The effect of intravenously infused noradrenaline [norepinephrine] upon the heart rate in man is principally mediated by:

Options for 115–116:

(A) a reflex decrease in parasympathetic discharge to the heart result ing from the change in mean arterial blood pressure
(B) a reflex increase in parasympathetic discharge to the heart result ing from the change in mean arterial blood pressure
(C) a reflex increase in sympathetic discharge to the heart resulting from the change in mean arterial blood pressure
(D) interaction of the drug with cardiac β-adrenoceptors

117 Select a potent antagonist of the effects of adrenaline [epinephrine upon pulse rate and upon peripheral resistance. The selected agen should be more potent against heart rate effects than against effect upon peripheral resistance.
118 Select a potent antagonist of the effects of adrenaline [epinephrine upon heart rate and upon peripheral resistance. The selected agen should be approximately equi-effective in each circumstance.

Options for 117–118:

ADR, α, & β

(A) phentolamine
(B) propranolol β-blocker
(C) salbutamol
(D) practolol
(E) phenoxybenzamine

Figure 6 represents the selectivity of action of directly acting sympathomime tic agents. Position A, at one extreme, represents a drug with agonist activity confined to α-adrenoceptors. Position D, at the other extreme, represents one with agonist activity confined to β-adrenoceptors. Indicate the position of the following drugs in *Figure 6*:

119 salbutamol
120 adrenaline [epinephrine]
121 methoxamine
122 isoprenaline [isoproterenol]
123 phenylephrine
124 orciprenaline [metaproterenol]

Options for 119–124:

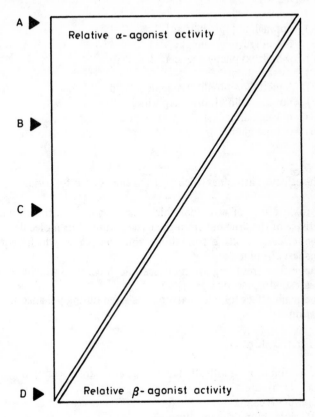

Figure 6

For each substrate and enzyme pair select the compound which is the major product of their interaction:

	Substrate +	Enzyme
125	3,4-dihydroxymandelic acid	catechol-*O*-methyltransferase
126	dopamine	dopamine β-oxidase
127	noradrenaline [norepinephrine]	catechol-*O*-methyltransferase
128	noradrenaline [norepinephrine]	monoamine oxidase
129	noradrenaline [norepinephrine]	phenylethanolamine *N*-methyltransferase
130	normetadrenaline [normetanephrine]	monoamine oxidase
131	tyramine	dopamine β-oxidase
132	tyramine	monoamine oxidase

Options for 125–132:

    (A)   adrenaline [epinephrine]
    (B)   3,4-dihydroxymandelic acid
    (C)   *p*-hydroxyphenylacetic acid
    (D)   metaraminol
    (E)   3-methoxy-4-hydroxymandelic acid
    (F)   noradrenaline [norepinephrine]
    (G)   normetadrenaline [normetanephrine]
    (H)   octopamine

Select the effect of atropine which best fits each of the following descriptions:

133 A toxic effect of atropine which results not from the antimuscarinic activity of the drug but from the basic nature of its molecule

134 The effect, resulting from muscarinic blockade, which requires the smallest atropine dosage

135 The effect, resulting from muscarinic blockade, which requires the greatest atropine dosage

136 The main effect for which atropine is given during pre-anaesthetic medication

Options for 133–136:

    (A)   inhibition of salivation and respiratory tract secretion
    (B)   tachycardia
    (C)   bradycardia
    (D)   inhibition of micturition
    (E)   inhibition of gastric oxyntic cell (HCl) secretion
    (F)   histamine release
    (G)   constipation
    (H)   dilation of the pupil

A full ganglion-blocking dose of pentolinium is administered subcutaneously to a resting healthy young man who is in a reclining position. How are each of the following changed by the administration of pentolinium:

137 The ability to focus the eye on a very distant object
138 The pupil diameter
139 The tone of the propulsive smooth muscle of the gut
140 The heart rate

Options for 137–140:

    (A) is increased
    (B) is reduced
    (C) is unchanged

For each of the patients select the one most suitable drug or combination of drugs with which the patient might be treated:

141 A soldier severely poisoned by the military gas sarin (an organophosphorus compound)
142 A child suffering from rapid-type mushroom poisoning (e.g. poisoning following ingestion of the red-staining inocybe)
143 An elderly woman in whom an attack of glaucoma has been precipitated by the injudicious use of cyclopentolate eyedrops
144 A depressed patient about to undergo electroconvulsive therapy
145 A patient remaining paralysed by pancuronium at the end of an operation

Options for 141–145

    (A) atropine
    (B) atropine and pralidoxime
    (C) suxamethonium [succinylcholine]
    (D) atropine and neostigmine
    (E) pilocarpine
    (F) a placebo containing dextrose

Select the one drug most likely to have produced each of the following patterns of responses when instilled into the eye:

	Pupil diameter	*Corneal touch reflex*	*Pupillary light reflex*	*Near point*
146	Increased	Present	Present	No change
147	Decreased	Present	Present	Decreased
148	Increased	Present	Absent	Increased
149	Increased	Absent	Present	No change

Options for 146–149:

(A) cocaine
(B) cyclopentolate
(C) phenylephrine
(D) pilocarpine
(E) procaine

In each of the following circumstances indicate the type of cardiac cell upon which the drug principally acts in order to produce its ameliorative effects:

150 The use of digoxin to correct a rapid ventricular rate due to atrial fibrillation
151 The use of propranolol to correct ventricular tachycardia due to a digoxin overdose
152 The use of digoxin to correct congestive heart failure with sinus rhythm
153 The use of atropine to correct sinus bradycardia evoked by the manipulation of abdominal viscera

Options for 150–153:

(A) cells of the sinoatrial node
(B) cells of the atrial myocardium
(C) cells of the atrioventricular node
(D) Purkinje cells
(E) cells of the ventricular myocardium

Three drugs X, Y and Z were each able to suppress twitches of the isolated rat diaphragm preparation elicited by stimulation of the phrenic nerve. The twitch suppression evoked by X, Y or Z was unaffected by the addition of choline to the bath fluid.

Concentrations of X, Y and Z which just suppressed twitches of the rat diaphragm elicited by phrenic nerve stimulation were also applied to the guinea-pig isolated ileum. Only drug X was observed to cause contraction of the ileum under these conditions. Drugs X and Y each caused contraction of the frog rectus abdominis muscle (multiply innervated skeletal muscle). Drug Z did not cause contraction of the rectus abdominis and did not antagonise the actions of X and Y upon this tissue.
Use this information for questions 154–156.

154 Drug X was:
155 Drug Y was:
156 Drug Z was:

Options for 154–156:

- (A) acetylcholine
- (B) botulinus toxin
- (C) gallamine
- (D) pancuronium
- (E) suxamethonium [succinylcholine]
- (F) tubocurarine
- (G) triethylcholine

Which phrase best describes the pharmacological properties of each of the following drug structures?

157

$$CH_3-\overset{\overset{\displaystyle CH_3}{|}}{\underset{\underset{\displaystyle CH_3}{|}}{N^+}}-CH_2-CH_2-CH_2-CH_2-CH_2-CH_2-\overset{\overset{\displaystyle CH_3}{|}}{\underset{\underset{\displaystyle CH_3}{|}}{N^+}}-CH_3$$

158

$$CH_3-\overset{\overset{\displaystyle CH_3}{|}}{\underset{\underset{\displaystyle CH_3}{|}}{N^+}}-CH_2-\overset{\overset{\displaystyle }{\underset{\underset{\displaystyle CH_3}{|}}{CH}}}{-}O-\overset{\overset{\displaystyle O}{\|}}{C}-CH_3$$

159

$$CH_3-\overset{\overset{\displaystyle CH_3}{|}}{\underset{\underset{\displaystyle CH_3}{|}}{N^+}}-CH_2-CH_2-O-\overset{\overset{\displaystyle O}{\|}}{C}-CH_2-CH_2-\overset{\overset{\displaystyle O}{\|}}{C}-O-CH_2-CH_2-\overset{\overset{\displaystyle CH_3}{|}}{\underset{\underset{\displaystyle CH_3}{|}}{N^+}}-CH_3$$

160

$$CH_3-\overset{\overset{\displaystyle CH_3}{|}}{\underset{\underset{\displaystyle CH_3}{|}}{N^+}}-CH_2-CH_2-O-\overset{\overset{\displaystyle O}{\|}}{C}-NH_2$$

161

$$CH_3-\overset{\overset{\displaystyle CH_3}{|}}{\underset{\underset{\displaystyle CH_3}{|}}{N^+}}-CH_2-CH_2-O-\overset{\overset{\displaystyle O}{\|}}{C}-CH_3$$

Options for 157–161:

(A) is the transmitter substance of cholinergic neurones
(B) is an agonist at the nicotinic cholinoceptors of skeletal muscle which is used clinically to produce brief periods of muscle paralysis
(C) is a potent agonist at muscarinic cholinoceptors but is relatively impotent as an agonist at nicotinic cholinoceptors
(D) is a potent agonist at both muscarinic and nicotinic cholinoceptors and is relatively resistant to hydrolysis by acetylcholinesterase
(E) is a competitive antagonist at the nicotinic cholinoceptors of skeletal muscle
(F) is a non-competitive antagonist at the nicotinic cholinoceptors of skeletal muscle
(G) is a competitive antagonist at the nicotinic cholinoceptors of autonomic ganglia
(H) is a non-competitive antagonist at the nicotinic cholinoceptors of autonomic ganglia

Indicate the undesirable side-effect which can accompany administration of the following drugs:

162 atropine (eyedrops) *muscarinic antag G*
163 neostigmine *Anti AChE   B*
164 guanethidine *ganglion blocker F*
165 propranolol *β-blocker D*
166 phenelzine *M, block B*

Options for 162–166:

(A) hyperplasia of the gums
(B) liver damage and a tendency to precipitate hypertensive crises
(C) bradycardia, excessive sweating and salivation
(D) precipitation of bronchoconstriction in susceptible patients
(E) gangrene of the extremities
(F) diarrhoea and failure of ejaculation
(G) precipitation of glaucoma in elderly patients
(H) fluorescent deposits in the primary dentition
(I) lesions of the cornea and peritoneum

A local anaesthetic drug has been allowed to equilibrate with an isolated neurone. When the neurone receives an appropriate stimulus it generates an action potential whose amplitude is smaller than that observed in the absence of the drug. Under these conditions, how are each of the following properties of the neurone modified by the presence of the drug?

167　The minimal stimulus strength required to elicit an action potential
168　The resting membrane potential of the neurone
169　The velocity of propagation of the action potential
170　The absolute refractory period of the neurone

Options for 167–170:

    (A)　is increased
    (B)　is unchanged
    (C)　is decreased

Type 6

171　(X)　The hydrolysis of methacholine by acetylcholinesterase
    (Y)　The hydrolysis of carbachol by acetylcholinesterase

172　(X)　The susceptibility of physiologically excited gastric oxyntic cells to muscarinic blockade
    (Y)　The susceptibility of physiologically excited eccrine sweat glands to muscarinic blockade

173　(X)　The nicotinic effects of carbachol
    (Y)　The nicotinic effects of methacholine

174　(X)　The normal refractory period of the atrioventricular node
    (Y)　The refractory period of the atrioventricular node after a therapeutic dose of digoxin

175　(X)　The normal refractory period of the atrioventricular node
    (Y)　The refractory period of the atrioventricular node after a therapeutic dose of propranolol

176　(X)　The slope of the cardiac pacemaker potential after noradrenaline [norepinephrine]
    (Y)　The slope of the cardiac pacemaker potential after methacholine

177　(X)　The rate of rise of the normal cardiac action potential
    (Y)　The rate of rise of the cardiac action potential after a therapeutic dose of lignocaine [lidocaine]

178 (X)   The α-agonist potency of methoxamine
     (Y)   The α-agonist potency of noradrenaline [norepinephrine]

179 (X)   The time required for noradrenergic neurone terminals to regain control noradrenaline [norepinephrine] concentrations after reserpine treatment
     (Y)   The time required for noradrenergic neurone cell bodies to regain control noradrenaline [norepinephrine] concentrations after reserpine treatment

180 (X)   The susceptibility of tyramine to biotransformation by monoamine oxidase
     (Y)   The susceptibility of amphetamine to biotransformation by monoamine oxidase

181 (X)   Alkylation of α-adrenoceptors by phenoxybenzamine
     (Y)   Alkylation of α-adrenoceptors by phenoxybenzamine when phentolamine is present

Type 9

182 The following compounds are substrates for the neuronal noradrenaline [norepinephrine] uptake mechanism and hence can gain access to the neuronal cytoplasm by that route:

     (A)   bethanidine
     (B)   ephedrine
     (C)   isoprenaline [isoproterenol]
     (D)   adrenaline [epinephrine]
     (E)   tyramine

183 α-adrenoceptors:

     (A)   mediate the relaxation of bronchial smooth muscle induced by phenylephrine
     (B)   are found in the propulsive smooth muscle of the gut and their activation results in inhibition of that tissue
     (C)   mediate the contraction of the dilator pupillae induced by cocaine eyedrops
     (D)   mediate the contraction of arteriolar smooth muscle induced by noradrenaline [norepinephrine]

184 The carbamoyl ester of choline (carbachol):

(A) increases the activity of the propulsive muscle of gut and bladder
(B) is rapidly inactivated by cholinesterase
(C) is an agonist at muscarinic cholinoceptors
(D) induces the release of adrenaline [epinephrine] from the adrenal medulla by activating nicotinic cholinoceptors

185 When a local anaesthetic is injected around a mixed bundle of nerve fibres:

(A) myelinated neurones of small diameter are anaesthetised before myelinated neurones of large diameter
(B) there is a minimum length for each nerve fibre which must be anaesthetised before action potential traffic through the area is prevented
(C) sensory (afferent) fibres are anaesthetised but motor (efferent) fibres are unaffected by the drug
(D) the sensation of sharp pain in the area subserved by the nerve bundle is lost before the sensation of firm pressure

186 The cardiac stimulant action of tyramine is:

(A) due to the release of noradrenaline [norepinephrine] from sympathetic nerves
(B) enhanced by cocaine
(C) enhanced by phenelzine
(D) antagonised by guanethidine
(E) antagonised by propranolol

187 β-adrenoceptors:

(A) are found in bronchiolar smooth muscle
(B) are found in intestinal smooth muscle, which also contains α-adrenoceptors
(C) mediate the increase in rate and force of cardiac contraction caused *in vitro* by tyramine
(D) mediate the increase in peripheral resistance in the splanchnic vascular bed due to efferent splanchnic nerve stimulation

188   The action of noradrenaline [norepinephrine], given by intravenous infusion to human subjects, on the heart rate:

   (A)   can be antagonised by either atropine or phentolamine
   (B)   after pretreatment with atropine, can be antagonised by propranolol
   (C)   after pretreatment with phentolamine, can be antagonised by propranolol
   (D)   after pretreatment with propranolol, cannot be antagonised by either atropine or phentolamine

189   Procaine:

   (A)   is an ester of *p*-aminobenzoic acid
   (B)   is often mixed with a vasoconstrictor agent in order to prolong its local anaesthetic action
   (C)   is suitable for use in topical anaesthesia
   (D)   is suitable for use in infiltration anaesthesia
   (E)   is suitable for use in epidural anaesthesia

190   Local anaesthetics, when injected around a nerve:

   (A)   prevent sudden changes in membrane permeability to both sodium and potassium ions
   (B)   increase the resting membrane potential
   (C)   affect small myelinated fibres earlier than large ones
   (D)   stabilise cell membranes most effectively when in the cationic form

191   Edrophonium:

   (A)   is a competitive inhibitor of acetylcholinesterase
   (B)   aids in the diagnosis of myasthenia gravis
   (C)   combines with the anionic site of the active centre of acetylcholinesterase
   (D)   combines with the esteratic site of the active centre of acetylcholinesterase

192 Neostigmine:

   (A) is a competitive inhibitor of acetylcholinesterase
   (B) is used in the treatment of myasthenia gravis
   (C) combines with the anionic site of the active centre of acetyl-
        cholinesterase
   (D) does not combine with the esteratic site of the active centre
        of acetylcholinesterase

193 Ecothiopate [echothiophate]:

   (A) is a non-competitive inhibitor of acetylcholinesterase
   (B) is used in the treatment of chronic simple (open angle) glaucoma
   (C) inhibits pseudocholinesterase more readily than acetylcholines-
        terase
   (D) does not combine with the anionic site of the active centre of
        acetylcholinesterase

194 Dyflos:

   (A) is a non-competitive inhibitor of acetylcholinesterase
   (B) can produce chronic neurotoxic effects including axonal destruc-
        tion and demyelination
   (C) inhibits pseudocholinesterase more readily than acetylcholines-
        terase
   (D) combines with both the anionic and the esteratic sites of the
        active centre of acetylcholinesterase

195 Pyridostigmine:

   (A) is a competitive inhibitor of acetylcholinesterase
   (B) is used to reverse the neuromuscular blocking action of suxa-
        methonium [succinylcholine]
   (C) is used in the treatment of myasthenia gravis
   (D) produces an inhibition of acetylcholinesterase which is indepen-
        dent of pH

196 Atropine:

   (A) reduces the effects of parasympathetic nerve activity on the urin-
        ary bladder more readily than it reduces the effects of sympa-
        thetic nerve activity on the eccrine sweat glands

(B) can reduce the effects of efferent vagal nerve activity on the heart and thereby induce tachycardia

(C) can stimulate the medullary vagal centre and thereby induce bradycardia

(D) is used in the treatment of rapid-type mushroom poisoning

197 Atropine:

(A) can cause photophobia when instilled into the eye

(B) can precipitate glaucoma when instilled into the eyes of elderly patients

(C) when instilled into the eye, improves the ability to focus on a very near object

(D) can cause the release of histamine from mast cells

198 Suxamethonium [succinylcholine]:

(A) when administered by intravenous injection induces fasciculation and then flaccid paralysis of focally innervated skeletal muscle

(B) is used to minimise the muscular component of the convulsion induced by electroconvulsive therapy

(C) is an antagonist at the nicotinic cholinoceptors of skeletal muscle

(D) causes contraction of multiply innervated skeletal muscle

199 Tubocurarine:

(A) is used in the treatment of severe strychnine intoxication

(B) is used in the treatment of botulism

(C) can cause the release of histamine from mast cells

(D) antagonises the contraction of multiply innervated skeletal muscle induced by carbachol

200 Carbachol:

(A) can cause the release of noradrenaline [norepinephrine] from postganglionic sympathetic neurones

(B) is used to treat postoperative atony of the gut

(C) is readily hydrolysed by acetylcholinesterase

(D) can prevent cholinergic transmission in autonomic ganglia

201 Pilocarpine:

(A) is an agonist at muscarinic cholinoceptors
(B) is used to produce a rapid lowering of intraocular pressure in acute congestive (narrow angle) glaucoma
(C) causes an increase in pupil diameter when instilled into the eye
(D) causes accommodation for near vision when instilled into the eye

2 Endocrine Pharmacology

including digoxin, diuretics and anticoagulants

Type 1

202 The concurrent administration of phenobarbitone increases the dose of warfarin required for effective anticoagulant therapy because:

(A) phenobarbitone displaces warfarin from albumin binding sites, thus increasing the rate of elimination of warfarin
(B) phenobarbitone forms an inactive complex with warfarin
(C) phenobarbitone induces liver microsomal oxidase, thus increasing the rate of biotransformation of warfarin
(D) phenobarbitone diminishes the renal tubular reabsorption of warfarin

203 The likelihood of digoxin-induced excessive cardiac excitability is increased by:

(A) high extracellular K^+ concentration
(B) low extracellular Ca^{2+} concentration
(C) low extracellular K^+ concentration
(D) high extracellular Mg^{2+} concentration

204 The oral anticoagulants (e.g. warfarin), in therapeutic doses, exert their main action by:

(A) reducing the plasma Ca^{2+} concentration
(B) preventing platelet aggregation
(C) preventing the action of thrombin

(D) inhibiting the synthesis of prothrombin through antagonism of vitamin K

205 Phytomenadione [phytonadione] is used therapeutically to overcome haemorrhage due to:

(A) dipyridamole
(B) heparin
(C) streptokinase
(D) warfarin

206 The clinically significant anticoagulant effects of warfarin are enhanced by phenylbutazone because:

(A) phenylbutazone itself has anticoagulant properties
(B) there is inhibition of liver metabolising enzymes
(C) there is competition for plasma protein binding sites
(D) there is competition for renal secretion

207 Heparin:

(A) is active *in vivo* only
(B) inhibits the conversion of prothrombin to thrombin
(C) antagonises vitamin K
(D) is active orally

208 A diuretic which acts as a competitive antagonist to aldosterone is:

(A) triamterene
(B) spironolactone
(C) metyrapone
(D) amiloride

209 The therapeutically most important action of cardiac glycosides when used in heart failure associated with normal rhythm is:

(A) sensitisation of carotid baroreceptors and increased vagal tone
(B) increased force of myocardial contraction
(C) stabilisation of cell membranes
(D) sensitisation of cardiac cells to acetylcholine

210   ADH (antidiuretic hormone):

(A)   is released from the anterior pituitary
(B)   is released in response to plasma hypotonicity
(C)   normally influences the kidney tubule to produce hypertonic urine
(D)   release is increased by high plasma ethanol concentrations

211   The daily synthesis of hydrocortisone by the human adrenal cortex is approximately:

(A)   0.25 mg
(B)   2.5 mg
(C)   25 mg
(D)   250 mg

212   In order to test anterior pituitary function, synthesis of adrenal corticosteroids may be blocked at the 11-deoxy stage by:

(A)   spironolactone
(B)   metyrapone
(C)   methisazone
(D)   cyproterone

213   The cardiac glycosides, in toxic doses, produce ventricular arrhythmias by an action on the:

(A)   sinoatrial node
(B)   atrial myocardium
(C)   atrioventricular node
(D)   Purkinje fibres
(E)   ventricular myocardium

214   The biguanide compound phenformin:

(A)   stimulates pancreatic A-cells (α-cells)
(B)   stimulates pancreatic B-cells (β-cells)
(C)   increases the absorption of glucose from the gut
(D)   promotes the uptake of glucose by muscle
(E)   decreases insulin sensitivity

215 The posterior pituitary secretes two hormones, both nonapeptides; one
is oxytocin, the other is:

(A) gonadotrophin
(B) antidiuretic hormone
(C) neurophysin
(D) prolactin
(E) inhibin

216 Metyrapone:

(A) is a synthetic corticosteroid
(B) when used as a diagnostic test will increase serum adrenocortico-
trophic hormone concentrations   ACTH
(C) secretion is increased by lysine vasopressin
(D) decreases plasma corticosteroid concentrations by a direct action
upon the central nervous system

Type 2

Which substance best fits each description? (applies to Questions 217–244)

217 It suppresses the release of chemical mediators arising from the antigen/
antibody reaction of anaphylaxis
218 It inhibits prostaglandin synthetase
219 It is a polypeptide with vasoconstrictor and bronchoconstrictor properties
220 It is a polypeptide with vasodilator and bronchoconstrictor properties
221 It is a surmountable antagonist when this acts to increase gastric secretion evoked by histamine

Options for 217–221:

(A) acetylsalicylic acid
(B) aldosterone
(C) angiotensin
(D) bradykinin
(E) cimetidine
(F) prostaglandin E_2
(G) sodium cromoglycate [cromolyn sodium]

222 Reduces the 'triple response' evoked by scratching histamine into the skin

223 An organic acid with anticoagulant properties released during mast cell degranulation

224 A monoamine found physiologically in blood platelets

225 Formed *in vivo* from arachidonic acid and is a potent stimulant of uterine smooth muscle and inhibitor of gastric secretion

226 an antagonist at 5-hydroxytryptamine D-receptors

Options for 222–226:

(A)   cimetidine
(B)   heparin
(C)   5-hydroxytryptamine
(D)   mepyramine
(E)   methysergide
(F)   prostaglandin E_2
(G)   renin
(H)   sodium cromoglycate [cromolyn sodium]

227 A β-globulin formed in the liver which requires vitamin K for its synthesis

228 An albumin with enzymic properties which catalyses the conversion of fibrinogen to fibrin

229 An anticoagulant which reduces the formation of prothrombin

230 An anticoagulant which reduces platelet adhesiveness

231 A compound which may be effective in correcting haemorrhage induced by streptokinase

Options for 227–231:

(A)   ε-aminocaproic acid
(B)   dipyridamole
(C)   fibrinolysin
(D)   heparin
(E)   prothrombin
(F)   thrombin
(G)   warfarin

232 A substance with a plasma half-life of about 40 min, which is degraded in the liver by a cleavage of disulphide bonds

233 A substance which will reverse hyperglycaemia in pancreatectomised animals

234 A substance producing a surge of insulin from the pancreas which cannot be repeated in less than 4 hours

235 A substance with an unknown mechanism of action, which does not stimulate pancreatic B-cells but requires trace amounts of insulin to increase the uptake and oxidation of glucose by fat tissues

Options for 232–235:

(A) alloxan
(B) insulin
(C) phenformin
(D) somatostatin
(E) tolbutamide

236 Inhibits Na^+ reabsorption in the distal tubule and also possesses weak carbonic anhydrase inhibitory properties

237 Inhibits Na^+ reabsorption mainly in the loop of Henle

238 Markedly inhibits HCO_3^- reabsorption and may cause a metabolic acidosis as a result

239 Inhibits the Na^+/K^+ 'exchange' in the distal tubule but does not act by antagonising aldosterone

240 Inhibits the Na^+/K^+ 'exchange' in the distal tubule through antagonism of aldosterone

Options for 236–240:

(A) acetazolamide
(B) amiloride
(C) bendrofluazide [bendroflumethiazide]
(D) ethacrynic acid
(E) spironolactone

241 A local hormone which causes increased capillary permeability, bronchiolar constriction and a marked stimulation of gastric acid secretion

242 A local hormone which causes increased capillary permeability, peripheral vasodilation and contraction of the pregnant uterus

243 A polypeptide local hormone which causes increased capillary permeability, bronchiolar constriction and relaxation of vascular smooth muscle

244 A polypeptide which causes marked vasoconstriction and stimulates the adrenal cortex to release aldosterone

Options for 241–244:

- (A)   angiotensin
- (B)   bradykinin
- (C)   gastrin
- (D)   histamine
- (E)   noradrenaline [norepinephrine]
- (F)   prostaglandin E_2

Type 3

In questions 245–251 answer:

- (A)   if response can be blocked by mepyramine alone
- (B)   if response can be blocked by cimetidine alone
- (C)   if response can be blocked only by a combination of mepyramine and cimetidine
- (D)   if response cannot be blocked by either mepyramine or cimetidine, alone or in combination

245   The release of histamine from tissue mast cells caused by morphine

246   The fall in blood pressure after intravenous injection of histamine

247   The oedema associated with Lewis's triple response

248   The acute inflammatory response to thermal injury

249   The increase in gastric secretion evoked by pentagastrin

250   The bronchoconstriction resulting from the antigen/antibody reaction of anaphylaxis

251   The pain after application of histamine to a blister base

In questions 252–255 answer:

- (A)   if the response can be blocked by methysergide alone
- (B)   if the response can be blocked by morphine alone
- (C)   if the response can be blocked only by a combination of methysergide and morphine
- (D)   if the response cannot be blocked by either methysergide or morphine, alone or in combination

252   The stimulant effect of 5-hydroxytryptamine on bronchial smooth muscle

253   The stimulant effect of 5-hydroxytryptamine on guinea-pig ileum

254 Bronchoconstriction resulting from the antigen/antibody reaction of anaphylaxis

255 Skin 'flushing' associated with cancer of the 5-hydroxytryptamine-producing cells of the intestine

In questions 256–259 answer:

   (A) if the statement applies to aspirin alone
   (B) if the statement applies to paracetamol [acetaminophen] alone
   (C) if the statement applies to both aspirin and paracetamol [acetaminophen]
   (D) if the statement applies to neither aspirin nor paracetamol [acetaminophen]

256 Antipyretic but not anti-inflammatory
257 Contraindicated in patients with peptic ulcer
258 Analgesic effects reversed by naloxone
259 Inhibits brain prostaglandin synthetase

Type 5

(260) belongs to a group of diuretics known as 'high ceiling' diuretics. Members of this group exert their major action in the (261), where they reduce (262). There is also a minor action reducing Na^+ reabsorption in (263). A clinical problem often associated with their long-term use is (264).

Options for 260–264:

260 (A) acetazolamide
     (B) chlorothiazide
     (C) frusemide [furosemide]
     (D) spironolactone

261 (A) ascending limb of loop of Henle
     (B) descending limb of loop of Henle
     (C) distal tubule
     (D) proximal tubule

262 (A) active HCO_3^- reabsorption
     (B) active Cl^- reabsorption
     (C) active K^+ reabsorption
     (D) active Na^+ reabsorption

263   (A)   ascending limb of loop of Henle
      (B)   descending limb of loop of Henle
      (C)   distal tubule
      (D)   proximal tubule

264   (A)   reduced plasma HCO_3^- concentration
      (B)   reduced plasma K^+ concentration
      (C)   reduced plasma Na^+ concentration
      (D)   reduced plasma uric acid concentration

Digoxin is effective in cardiac failure with sinus rhythm because it produces (265). If however there is atrial fibrillation, digoxin controls the associated tachycardia by a direct action at the (266). The most frequent cause of death from digoxin intoxication is (267), an effect of digoxin on the (268). This is more likely to occur in the presence of (269).

Options for 265–269:

265   (A)   sensitisation of carotid baroreceptors and increased vagal tone
      (B)   increased force of myocardial contraction
      (C)   stabilisation of cell membranes
      (D)   sensitisation of cardiac cells to acetylcholine

266   (A)   sinoatrial node
      (B)   atrial myocardium
      (C)   atrioventricular node
      (D)   Purkinje fibres
      (E)   ventricular myocardium

267   (A)   atrial flutter
      (B)   atrial fibrillation
      (C)   complete atrioventricular block
      (D)   ventricular fibrillation

268   (A)   sinoatrial node
      (B)   atrial myocardium
      (C)   atrioventricular node
      (D)   Purkinje fibres
      (E)   ventricular myocardium

269   (A)   low extracellular Ca^{2+} concentration
      (B)   high extracellular Mg^{2+} concentration
      (C)   low extracellular K^+ concentration
      (D)   low extracellular Na^+ concentration

istamine is a powerful stimulant of (270) secretion. Parietal gland cells are
imulated to give (271) and (272) gland cells are stimulated to give pepsino-
n. Like (273) this action of histamine is mediated by combination with
274) receptors and can therefore be selectively antagonised by (275).

ptions for 270–275:

70　(A)　sweat
　　(B)　gastric
　　(C)　insulin
　　(D)　bronchial

71　(A)　pentagastrin
　　(B)　insulin
　　(C)　pepsinogen
　　(D)　hydrochloric acid

72　(A)　peptic
　　(B)　β
　　(C)　parotid
　　(D)　mucous

73　(A)　bronchiolar constriction
　　(B)　cardiac stimulation
　　(C)　intestinal contraction
　　(D)　vasodilation

274　(A)　H_1
　　(B)　H_2
　　(C)　nicotinic
　　(D)　β

275　(A)　cimetidine
　　(B)　cyproheptidine
　　(C)　mepyramine
　　(D)　propranolol

(276) belongs to a group of relatively weak diuretics used for their ability to
conserve (277). The site of this action is the (278). (279) also has the ability
to conserve (277) but unlike (276) the action is exerted by (280).

Options for 276–280:

276 (A) acetazolamide
(B) amiloride
(C) ethacrynic acid
(D) frusemide [furosemide]

277 (A) bicarbonate ions
(B) chloride ions
(C) hydrogen ions
(D) potassium ions

278 (A) ascending limb of loop of Henle
(B) descending limb of loop of Henle
(C) distal tubule
(D) proximal tubule

279 (A) chlorothiazide
(B) ethacrynic acid
(C) spironolactone
(D) triamterene

280 (A) inhibition of angiotensin formation
(B) direct inhibition of aldosterone synthesis
(C) induction of aldosterone-metabolising enzymes
(D) competitive antagonism of aldosterone

Two groups of rats were injected with (281) which selectively destroys t
(282), inducing an experimental state of (283). Several days later, the ra
were noticed to have diuresis accompanied by (284), which causes the ur
ary excretion of large amounts of (285). One group of rats was treated w
tolbutamide, the other group with insulin. The animals treated with tolbu
mide survived for (286) those treated with insulin.

Options for 281–286:

281 (A) alloxan
(B) chlorpropamide
(C) phenformin
(D) tolbutamide

282 (A) A-cells of the pancreas
(B) B-cells of the pancreas

(C) A- and B-cells of the pancreas
(D) exocrine cells of the pancreas

283 (A) diabetes mellitus
(B) diabetes insipidus
(C) hypoglycaemia
(D) polyneuritis

284 (A) hyperglycaemia
(B) hypoglycaemia
(C) glycosuria
(D) polyneuritis

285 (A) glucose
(B) insulin
(C) ketone bodies
(D) urea

286 (A) a shorter time than
(B) a longer time than
(C) a similar time to

(287) is an anticoagulant which is given to man only by injection. It produces its anticoagulant effect primarily by (288). It is antagonised by (289). (290), an oral anticoagulant also used as a rodenticide, produces its anticoagulant effect by (291) and is antagonised by (292).

Options for 287–292:

287 (A) citrate
(B) dipyridamole
(C) heparin
(D) warfarin

288 (A) decreasing formation of prothrombin
(B) decreasing formation of thrombin
(C) preventing the action of thrombin
(D) reducing platelet adhesiveness

289 (A) vitamin K
(B) compounds with a high positive charge
(C) compounds with a high negative charge
(D) calcium ions

290 (A) citrate
    (B) dipyridamole
    (C) heparin
    (D) warfarin

291 (A) decreasing formation of prothrombin
    (B) decreasing formation of thrombin
    (C) preventing the action of thrombin
    (D) reducing platelet adhesiveness

292 (A) vitamin K
    (B) compounds with a high positive charge
    (C) compounds with a high negative charge
    (D) calcium ions

(293), the principal hormone secreted by the thyroid gland, makes up (294) of the organically bound iodine in the thyroid venous blood. Its secretion from the gland is stimulated physiologically by (295), which is released from the (296) in response to changes in the free blood concentration of (297). A decline in thyroid hormone secretion can be produced by administration of (298), an antithyroid agent which inhibits the active uptake of iodide by the gland.

Options for 293–298:

293 (A) diiodotyrosine
    (B) thyroglobulin
    (C) thyroxine
    (D) triiodothyronine

294 (A) 10%
    (B) 40%
    (C) 60%
    (D) 90%

295 (A) long-acting thyroid stimulator
    (B) thyroglobulin
    (C) thyrotrophic hormone
    (D) thyroxine-binding globulin

296 (A) anterior pituitary gland
    (B) posterior pituitary gland
    (C) hypothalamus
    (D) thalamus

297 (A) diiodotyrosine
    (B) iodide
    (C) iodine
    (D) thyroid hormone

298 (A) carbimazole
    (B) ^{131}I
    (C) potassium iodide
    (D) potassium perchlorate

(299) and (300) are two of the most important hormones secreted by the adrenal cortex. The synthesis and release of (299) is stimulated by (301) whereas that of (300) is stimulated by (302) which also constricts the blood vessels. The actions of the adrenal steroids can be divided into two categories, glucocorticoid and mineralocorticoid; at pharmacological doses (299) possesses (303) activity and (300) possesses (304) activity.

Options for 299–304:

299 (A) aldosterone
    (B) cortisone
    (C) deoxycorticosterone
    (D) hydrocortisone

300 (A) aldosterone
    (B) hydrocortisone
    (C) progesterone
    (D) spironolactone

301 (A) adrenocorticotrophic hormone
    (B) follicle-stimulating hormone
    (C) luteinising hormone
    (D) thyroid-stimulating hormone

302 (A) angiotensin
    (B) bradykinin
    (C) kallidin
    (D) prostaglandin E_1

303 (A) mainly glucocorticoid
and (B) mainly mineralocorticoid
304 (C) glucocorticoid and significant mineralocorticoid

(305) is a substance released from the kidney in response to decrease in blood volume. This substance brings about the formation of (306) from its inactive precursor (307). (306), as well as acting on the renal vessels, acts on the adrenal cortex to increase the output of (308). This in turn acts on the kidney to (309).

Options for 305–309:

305 (A)   angiotensin
     (B)   angiotensinogen
     (C)   renin
     (D)   rennin

306 (A)   angiotensin
     (B)   angiotensinogen
     (C)   bradykinin
     (D)   vasopressin

307 (A)   angiotensin
     (B)   angiotensinogen
     (C)   bradykinin
     (D)   bradykininogen

308 (A)   aldosterone
     (B)   hydrocortisone
     (C)   metyrapone
     (D)   prednisolone

309 (A)   increase Na^+ and K^+ reabsorption
     (B)   increase Na^+ reabsorption, decrease K^+ reabsorption
     (C)   decrease Na^+ reabsorption, increase K^+ reabsorption
     (D)   decrease Na^+ and K^+ reabsorption

Type 6   A = X > Y
               B = X = Y
               C = X < Y

310 (X)   percentage of an oral dose of prednisolone found in plasma
     (Y)   percentage of an oral dose of deoxycorticosterone found in plasma

311 (X)   the Na^+ retaining action of fludrocortisone
     (Y)   the Na^+ retaining action of betamethasone

312 (X) time between vitamin K administration and antagonism of warfarin-induced haemorrhage

(Y) time between whole blood transfusion and antagonism of warfarin-induced haemorrhage

313 (X) influence of plasma aldosterone concentration on ACTH (adrenocorticotrophic hormone) output

(Y) influence of plasma hydrocortisone concentration on ACTH output

314 (X) aldosterone secretion in presence of low plasma Na^+ concentration

(Y) aldosterone secretion in presence of raised plasma Na^+ concentration

315 (X) plasma half-life of thyroxine

(Y) plasma half-life of triiodothyronine

316 (X) basal metabolic rate of a normal animal

(Y) basal metabolic rate of an animal treated with carbimazole

317 (X) plasma aldosterone concentrations after treatment with spironolactone

(Y) plasma aldosterone concentrations after treatment with metyrapone

318 (X) the cardiotoxic effects of digoxin in the presence of decreased extracellular Ca^{2+} concentration

(Y) the cardiotoxic effects of digoxin in the presence of increased extracellular Ca^{2+} concentration

319 (X) thyrotrophin secretion in normal animals

(Y) thyrotrophin secretion in animals pretreated with thyroxine

320 (X) dose of radioactive iodide to diagnose hyperthyroidism

(Y) dose of radioactive iodide to treat hyperthyroidism

321 (X) the rate of uptake by the thyroid gland of radioactive iodide

(Y) the rate of uptake by the thyroid gland of unlabelled iodide

322 (X) rate of uptake of iodide by the thyroid gland after treatment with carbimazole

(Y) rate of uptake of iodide by the thyroid gland after treatment with potassium perchlorate

323 (X) the cardiotoxic effects of digoxin in the presence of decreased extracellular K^+ concentration

(Y) the cardiotoxic effects of digoxin in the presence of increased extracellular K^+ concentration

324 (X) anti-inflammatory potency of dexamethasone
(Y) the Na^+ retaining potency of dexamethasone

325 (X) anti-inflammatory potency of aldosterone
(Y) anti-inflammatory potency of hydrocortisone

326 (X) central venous pressure in patient with normal cardiac function
(Y) central venous pressure in patient with cardiac failure

327 (X) the concentration of insulin in the plasma of a diabetic patient 12 hours after injection of 40 units of soluble insulin

(Y) the concentration of insulin in the plasma of a diabetic patient 12 hours after injection of 40 units of crystalline zinc insulin

328 (X) peak plasma concentration of insulin after 400 mg tolbutamide
(Y) peak plasma concentration of insulin after 800 mg tolbutamide

329 (X) plasma aldosterone concentration in untreated congestive heart failure

(Y) plasma aldosterone concentration in congestive heart failure under effective treatment with digoxin

330 (X) the anti-inflammatory action of aspirin
(Y) the anti-inflammatory action of paracetamol [acetaminophen]

331 (X) gastrointestinal blood loss caused by a 300 mg tablet of aspirin
(Y) gastrointestinal blood loss caused by a 500 mg tablet of paracetamol [acetaminophen]

332 (X) prostaglandin synthetase inhibitory activity of aspirin
(Y) prostaglandin synthetase inhibitory activity of paracetamol [acetaminophen]

Type 7

333 (X) plasma concentration of hydrocortisone
(Y) release of ACTH from the anterior pituitary gland

334 (X) circulating aldosterone concentration
(Y) kidney tubule fluid concentration of K^+

335 (X) plasma concentration of metyrapone
(Y) plasma concentration of hydrocortisone

336 (X) circulating thyroxine concentrations
(Y) release of thyroid-stimulating hormone from the anterior pituitary gland

337 (X) plasma concentration of carbimazole
(Y) ability of thyroid gland to accumulate iodide actively

Type 8

338 Mepyramine blocks the stimulant effects of a histamine aerosol on bronchial smooth muscle

BECAUSE

mepyramine dilates bronchial smooth muscle

339 Cimetidine inhibits gastric secretion evoked by histamine

BECAUSE

cimetidine is an antagonist at histamine H_2 receptors

340 Prostaglandin E_2 is used for therapeutic termination of pregnancy

BECAUSE

prostaglandin E_2 stimulates uterine muscle to contract in early pregnancy

341 Ergotamine is used in the treatment of migraine

BECAUSE

ergotamine is a 5-hydroxytryptamine D-receptor antagonist

342   Morphine can cause skin irritation and itching

BECAUSE

morphine releases histamine from tissue mast cells

343   Pentagastrin is preferred to histamine for tests of gastric function

BECAUSE

pentagastrin, unlike histamine, has no circulatory actions

344   Angiotensin increases systemic blood pressure immediately after intravenous injection

BECAUSE

angiotensin releases aldosterone from the adrenal cortex

345   Antihistamine creams may cause skin irritation

BECAUSE

antihistamines applied to the skin are potent allergens

346   Cimetidine blocks the stimulant effects of a histamine aerosol on bronchial smooth muscle

BECAUSE

cimetidine is an antagonist at histamine H_2 receptors

347   Sodium cromoglycate [cromolyn sodium] is administered by inhalation in asthma

BECAUSE

in asthma the site of action of sodium cromoglycate is the bronchial tree

348 Bendrofluazide [bendroflumethiazide] may produce hyponatraemia

BECAUSE

bendrofluazide inhibits reabsorption of Na^+ in the proximal tubule

349 Acetazolamide produces a self-limiting alkalosis

BECAUSE

acetazolamide inhibits the activity of carbonic anhydrase

350 Gout is a possible side-effect of treatment with ethacrynic acid

BECAUSE

ethacrynic acid competes with uric acid for excretion

351 Sodium cromoglycate [cromolyn sodium] is effective clinically in allergic asthma

BECAUSE

sodium cromoglycate inhibits antibody formation by the reticuloendothelial system

352 Triamterene increases sodium reabsorption (associated with potassium excretion) in the kidney

BECAUSE

triamterene is an aldosterone antagonist

353 Frusemide [furosemide] may provoke digitalis intoxication

BECAUSE

frusemide decreases the excretion of K^+ by the kidney

354   In young children and pregnancy ^{132}I is preferred in diagnostic tests for thyroid malfunction

BECAUSE

^{132}I has a long half-life and emits only γ-rays

355   The thiazide diuretics may provoke digitalis intoxication

BECAUSE

the thiazide diuretics increase K^+ loss by the kidney

356   Protamine sulphate may be used to counteract haemorrhage due to heparin overdosage

BECAUSE

protamine is a low molecular weight protein with a high net positive charge

357   Paracetamol [acetaminophen] has powerful anti-inflammatory properties

BECAUSE

paracetamol inhibits brain prostaglandin synthetase in concentrations obtained clinically

358   Diphenhydramine is used clinically to combat motion sickness

BECAUSE

diphenhydramine blocks responses to histamine mediated through H_1 receptors

359   Concomitant administration of barbiturates may reduce the effectiveness of the oral anti-coagulants, e.g. warfarin

BECAUSE

the barbiturates induce increased formation of metabolising enzymes by the liver

360 The sulphonylurea oral hypoglycaemic agents
are of value in juvenile diabetes

BECAUSE

the pancreatic B-cells in juvenile diabetes are
unable to secrete insulin

361 Glibenclamide lowers blood glucose concentration
more rapidly than other sulphonylureas

BECAUSE

glibenclamide enhances insulin's ability to promote
the uptake of glucose into tissues

Type 9

362 Angiotensin:

    (A)   stimulates the adrenal cortex to release aldosterone
    (B)   has a short (1–2 min) half-life in plasma
    (C)   is a chemical mediator of acute inflammation
    (D)   is a potent peripheral vasoconstrictor agent
    (E)   is formed by the action of renin on plasma α-globulin

363 Both bradykinin and prostaglandin E_2:

    (A)   dilate peripheral blood vessels
    (B)   are polypeptides formed from plasma α-globulins
    (C)   increase vascular permeability
    (D)   cause pain when applied to a blister base
    (E)   are likely mediators of acute inflammation

364 5-hydroxytryptamine D-receptors:

    (A)   are blocked by phenoxybenzamine
    (B)   mediate bronchoconstrictor responses evoked by 5-hydroxy-tryptamine
    (C)   are stimulated and blocked by lysergic acid diethylamide (LSD)
    (D)   mediate the flushing of skin associated with carcinoid syndrome
    (E)   are blocked by methysergide

365   Tissue mast cells:

(A)   store histamine complexed with adenosine triphosphate (ATP)
(B)   can be depleted of their histamine by compound 48:80
(C)   release histamine and heparin during the antigen/antibody reactic
        of anaphylaxis
(D)   play a role in Lewis's Triple Response to scratching the skin
(E)   can be induced to release histamine by morphine

366   Both aspirin and indomethacin:

(A)   inhibit prostaglandin synthetase
(B)   suppress the later part of the acute inflammatory response (afte
        60 min)
(C)   inhibit the increased capillary permeability induced by bradykini
(D)   are anti-inflammatory and antipyretic
(E)   fail to suppress the antigen/antibody reaction of anaphylaxis

367   Sodium cromoglycate [cromolyn sodium] :

(A)   is poorly absorbed after oral administration
(B)   has neither anti-inflammatory nor bronchodilator activity
(C)   suppresses the response of a sensitised tissue to the antigen
(D)   antagonises   histamine-   and   bradykinin-induced   broncho
        constriction
(E)   suppresses histamine release from mast cells by compound 48:80

368   Triiodothyronine:

(A)   is transported in blood bound to an α-globulin
(B)   forms roughly 10% of the circulating form of thyroid hormone
(C)   is stored in the colloid of the thyroid gland as thyroglobulin
(D)   is useful in the treatment of exophthalmic goitre
(E)   is more potent than thyroxine on a mole-for-mole basis

369   In thyrotoxicosis:

(A)   uptake of ^{131}I by thyroid is diminished
(B)   the amount of iodine bound to serum protein is increased
(C)   the heart rate is increased
(D)   oxygen consumption is increased

370 Carbimazole:

    (A)   selectively blocks the incorporation (by the thyroid gland) of iodine into an organic molecule
    (B)   is useful in the treatment of hyperthyroidism
    (C)   selectively blocks iodide uptake by the thyroid gland
    (D)   decreases basal metabolic rate
    (E)   can produce goitre by increased secretion of thyrotrophin

371 Thyrotrophin secretion:

    (A)   occurs from the anterior lobe of the pituitary gland
    (B)   promotes the release of thyroid hormone from the thyroid gland
    (C)   is regulated in part by hypothalamic thyrotrophin-releasing factor
    (D)   is inhibited by high thyroxine blood concentrations
    (E)   is increased by long-acting thyroid stimulator

372 After total thyroidectomy:

    (A)   the blood concentration of thyrotrophin is decreased
    (B)   basal metabolic rate is decreased
    (C)   myxoedema develops
    (D)   the blood concentration of thyroid hormone is decreased
    (E)   the blood concentration of thyrotrophin-releasing factor is increased

373 Fibrinolysin (plasmin):

    (A)   is normally present in plasma
    (B)   can be antagonised by ε-aminocaproic acid
    (C)   breaks down clots to soluble products
    (D)   may cause haemorrhage

374 Citrate:

    (A)   is used to prevent stored blood from clotting
    (B)   is metabolised in the Krebs cycle
    (C)   prevents the formation of thrombin
    (D)   inhibits thromboplastin formation
    (E)   may be used *in vivo* as an anticoagulant

375 Dipyridamole:

    (A)   relaxes most smooth muscle
    (B)   is used in the treatment of angina pectoris
    (C)   interferes with the action of prothrombin
    (D)   reduces platelet aggregation and adhesion

376 Heparin:

    (A)   inhibits the conversion of prothrombin to thrombin
    (B)   inhibits platelet clumping
    (C)   has a high net positive charge in aqueous solution
    (D)   must be given parenterally in order to obtain an anticoagulant effect
    (E)   occurs naturally in mast cells complexed with protein

377 Warfarin:

    (A)   in the plasma is mostly protein bound
    (B)   decreases the formation of prothrombin
    (C)   may be potentiated by phenylbutazone
    (D)   is active both *in vivo* and *in vitro*

378 Acetazolamide:

    (A)   causes the bicarbonate concentration in the urine to rise
    (B)   produces a self-limiting alkalosis
    (C)   is active after oral administration
    (D)   causes bone marrow depression as a rare side-effect

379 ACTH

    (A)   is a polypeptide formed in the pituitary gland
    (B)   output is regulated in part by plasma aldosterone concentrations
    (C)   output is regulated in part by hypothalamic influences
    (D)   is used as a diagnostic aid in cases of adrenocortical insufficiency

380 Angiotensin:

(A) is an octapeptide derived from an inactive precursor in the plasma
(B) produces marked vasodilation, with a resultant fall in systolic and diastolic blood pressure
(C) stimulates the adrenal cortex to release aldosterone
(D) stimulates the adrenal medulla to release catecholamines

381 Pentagastrin:

(A) is a synthetic analogue of gastrin
(B) stimulates gastric acid secretion
(C) is used in tests of gastric function
(D) has circulatory actions similar to those of histamine

382 Frusemide [furosemide]:

(A) is active in the presence of acidosis or alkalosis
(B) inhibits Na^+ reabsorption mainly in the ascending limb of the loop of Henle
(C) produces a diuresis which is slow in onset and prolonged
(D) elevates plasma uric acid concentrations and may precipitate acute gout

383 Amiloride:

(A) interferes with the Na^+/K^+ 'exchange' in the distal tubule
(B) is a competitive antagonist of aldosterone
(C) may produce hyperkalaemia
(D) elevates plasma urea concentrations

384 Ethacrynic acid:

(A) produces a very marked diuresis of short duration
(B) elevates plasma uric acid concentrations and may precipitate gout
(C) is used for its ability to conserve K^+
(D) may produce circulatory collapse

385 Acetazolamide:

(A) inhibits the action of carbonic anhydrase
(B) produces an alkaline urine
(C) produces a self-limiting acidosis which may be corrected by ammonium chloride administration
(D) produces a marked loss of K^+

386 Thiazide diuretics:

(A) possess weak activity as inhibitors of carbonic anhydrase
(B) have an antihypertensive effect which is independent of their diuretic action
(C) elevate plasma uric acid concentrations and may precipitate gout
(D) are ineffective in the presence of a metabolic acidosis

387 The cardiotoxic effects of cardiac glycosides are increased by:

(A) high extracellular K^+ concentration
(B) high extracellular Ca^{2+} concentration
(C) low extracellular K^+ concentration
(D) low extracellular Mg^{2+} concentration

388 Spironolactone:

(A) blocks the synthesis of aldosterone
(B) decreases retention of Na^+ and water by the kidney
(C) is used as a diuretic particularly where excess aldosterone is implicated in the oedema
(D) decreases K^+ and H^+ loss

389 Possible side-effects from long-term treatment with anti-inflammatory corticosteroids include:

(A) suppression of ACTH output and adrenal atrophy
(B) lens cataract formation
(C) hypoglycaemia
(D) muscle wasting

390 Prothrombin:

(A) is a β-globulin formed in the liver
(B) requires vitamin K for synthesis
(C) catalyses the conversion of fibrinogen to fibrin
(D) is present in normal plasma before clotting commences

391 Fibrinogen:

(A) is a soluble globulin formed in the liver
(B) is converted to fibrin during the clotting process
(C) is present in normal plasma before clotting commences
(D) is broken down by fibrinolysin

392 Protamine sulphate:

(A) is a low molecular weight protein
(B) is strongly basic at body pH
(C) inhibits the thrombin/fibrinogen interaction
(D) is used in cases of heparin overdosage
(E) often produces a marked antigen/antibody reaction

393 Heparin:

(A) occurs naturally in the body
(B) plays a physiological role in the control of blood clotting
(C) prevents the action of thrombin
(D) must be administered parenterally
(E) prevents clotting both *in vivo* and *in vitro*

394 Sodium edetate (the disodium salt of ethylenediaminetetra-acetic acid):

(A) removes ionic calcium from the plasma
(B) is used *in vivo* to prevent thrombus formation
(C) slows the conversion of prothrombin to thrombin
(D) decreases the action of Factor XIII (fibrin-stabilising factor)

395   Warfarin:

    (A)   reduces the formation of Factors IX and X and prothrombin
    (B)   is active *in vivo* and *in vitro*
    (C)   may be less effective in a patient on regular barbiturate therapy
    (D)   may be potentiated by weak acids with a high affinity for plasma proteins
    (E)   can produce a haemorrhage which is overcome by vitamin K

396   The thioureas (e.g. carbimazole):

    (A)   interfere with the iodination of tyrosine
    (B)   are well absorbed from the intestine
    (C)   have a rapid onset of action
    (D)   may cause skin rashes and agranulocytosis

397   Tolbutamide:

    (A)   is absorbed after oral administration
    (B)   is metabolised by the liver
    (C)   is effective in juvenile diabetes
    (D)   is effective in maturity onset diabetes
    (E)   stimulates pancreatic B-cells to release insulin

398   Both aspirin and paracetamol [acetaminophen]:

    (A)   inhibit brain prostaglandin synthetase
    (B)   are antipyretic
    (C)   fail to suppress the antigen/antibody reaction of anaphylaxis
    (D)   are effective anti-inflammatory agents
    (E)   can bind to plasma protein

399   Carbimazole:

    (A)   is used prior to subtotal thyroidectomy
    (B)   is well absorbed from the intestine
    (C)   inhibits the thyroid iodide pump
    (D)   causes skin rashes

400 In hyperthyroidism:

(A) basal metabolic rate is increased
(B) sensitivity to catecholamines is increased
(C) heart rate, cardiac output and blood pressure are increased
(D) treatment is with thyroxine or triiodothyronine

401 In hypothyroidism:

(A) oxygen consumption is decreased
(B) treatment is with thyroxine
(C) sensitivity to catecholamines is increased
(D) intestinal activity decreases

402 Insulin is secreted by the B-cells of the pancreas into the blood:

(A) at a rate regulated by the blood glucose concentration
(B) in response to sulphonylurea compounds
(C) in response to biguanide compounds
(D) in subnormal amounts in growth-onset diabetes mellitus

403 Glucagon:

(A) causes breakdown of muscle glycogen
(B) increases blood glucose concentration
(C) is secreted by the A-cells of the pancreas
(D) inhibits insulin secretion by the pancreas

404 A helpful measurement for the diagnosis of Cushing's syndrome is the urinary output of 17-oxogenic steroids. Increased urinary output of 17-oxogenic steroids can be achieved in normal subjects by the administration of:

(A) insulin
(B) metyrapone
(C) lysine vasopressin
(D) tetracosactrin
(E) hydrocortisone

3 Reproductive Pharmacology

Type 1

405 Prostaglandin $F_{2\alpha}$ causes:

(A) an increase in progesterone secretion from corpora lutea
(B) an increase in oestradiol secretion from corpora lutea
(C) a decrease in progesterone secretion from corpora lutea
(D) a decrease in oestradiol secretion from corpora lutea

406 It is used as the oestrogenic component of some combined-type oral contraceptive agents:

(A) mestranol
(B) oestradiol
(C) oestrone
(D) norethisterone
(E) stilboestrol [diethylstilbestrol]

407 It has been suggested (Committee on Safety of Medicines, 1970) that the dose of oestrogen in oral contraceptives should be below which of the following values, if the incidence of thrombo-embolism is to be reduced:

(A) 500 μg
(B) 200 μg
(C) 100 μg
(D) 50 μg
(E) 20 μg
(F) 5 μg

408 The ratio of deaths in 1 year attributable to cigarette smoking compared to those attributable to oral contraceptives is of the order:

(A) 0.001 to 1
(B) 0.1 to 1
(C) 1 to 1
(D) 100 to 1
(E) 10 000 to 1

409 The stage of development, in spermatogenesis, after the spermatocyte is:

(A) spermatid
(B) spermatozoa
(C) spermatogonia

410 Development of the male genital tract will occur *in utero* in genetic females after giving the mother:

(A) dydrogesterone
(B) hydroxyprogesterone hexanoate
(C) chlormadinone acetate
(D) testosterone
(E) thalidomide

411 The low-dose, progestogen-only type of oral contraceptive acts by:

(A) inhibition of the midcycle surge of luteinising hormone secretion
(B) inhibition of follicle-stimulating hormone secretion
(C) preventing ovulation
(D) rendering cervical mucus hostile to sperm

412 Oxytocin is used therapeutically in humans to:

(A) maintain lactation
(B) initiate labour
(C) increase libido
(D) prevent conception
(E) induce abortion in the first trimester

413 Release of this hormone from the pituitary gland is inhibited by a hormone from the hypothalamus:

(A) prolactin
(B) corticotrophin
(C) luteinising hormone
(D) thyroid-stimulating hormone

414 The posterior pituitary gland is connected to the median eminence by the:

(A) thalamus
(B) vascular portal system
(C) connective tissue
(D) neural tracts
(E) sella turcica

415 Oxytocin is transported down the axons to the pituitary gland after being synthesised in the:

(A) premamillary nuclei
(B) supraoptic nuclei
(C) substantia nigra
(D) arcuate nuclei
(E) paraventricular nuclei

416 Drugs which interfere with neurotransmission in the brain can produce side-effects by altering prolactin release. Galactorrhoea may be produced by:

(A) physostigmine
(B) levodopa
(C) chlordiazepoxide
(D) chlorpromazine

417 Esterification of 17β-oestradiol and testosterone changes the pharmacological profile as it:

(A) makes the compound orally active
(B) prolongs the duration of action

(C) increases the chemical stability in the injection fluid
(D) produces a different spectrum of actions

18 Virilisation in the Stein–Leventhal syndrome is due to increased:

(A) testicular androgen secretion
(B) testicular oestrogen secretion
(C) ovarian androgen secretion
(D) ovarian oestrogen secretion
(E) adrenal corticosteroid secretion
(F) adrenal androgen secretion
(G) adrenal oestrogen secretion

19 Where there is a deficiency of Leydig-cell biosynthetic activity, the size and functioning of male secondary sexual organs can be maintained with:

(A) fluoxymesterone
(B) mestranol
(C) aetiocholanolone
(D) androsterone

20 This drug (or combination of drugs) is used to induce ovulation in cases of infertility associated with persistently low oestrogen secretions:

(A) ethinyloestradiol
(B) clomiphene
(C) bovine follicle-stimulating hormone then bovine luteinising hormone
(D) human postmenopausal gonadotrophin then human chorionic gonadotrophin
(E) ethinyloestradiol + norethisterone

21 The molecule which releases thyroid-stimulating hormone from the pituitary gland is considered to be:

(A) a glycoprotein
(B) a steroid
(C) a small peptide
(D) a protein

(E)   an adrenergic neurotransmitter
(F)   a cholinergic neurotransmitter

422   Which of the following compounds is used for treatment of all th
following conditions: severe debility, osteoporosis, convalescence afte
major surgery anaemias:

(A)   stilboestrol [diethylstilbestrol]
(B)   fluoxymesterone
(C)   norethisterone
(D)   cyproterone
(E)   nandrolone

423   Bromocriptine inhibits lactation by:

(A)   competitively antagonising oestrogens acting on the mammary
glands
(B)   inhibiting oxytocin release
(C)   antagonising prolactin acting on the mammary glands
(D)   inhibiting the secretion of prolactin

424   This inactive steroid is demethylated *in vivo* to form a steroid posses
ing oestrogenic activity:

(A)   oestradiol benzoate
(B)   stilboestrol [diethylstilbestrol]
(C)   mestranol
(D)   piperazine oestrone sulphate
(E)   ethinyloestradiol

425   A new drug injected into a prepubertal female rat produced an increas
in uterine weight. This action could be prevented by prior removal o
the ovaries. The drug was most likely to act as an:

(A)   agonist at oestrogen receptors
(B)   antagonist at oestrogen receptors
(C)   agonist at gonadotrophin receptors
(D)   agonist at progestogen receptors

426 A new drug injected into male rats produced immediate sterility. Its likely site of action was the:

(A) hypothalamus
(B) anterior pituitary gland
(C) seminiferous tubule
(D) epididymis

427 The androgenic/anabolic potency ratio relative to testosterone is greater than 1 in the case of:

(A) mesterolone
(B) stanozolol
(C) nandrolone
(D) methandienone

428 Reversible intrahepatic obstructive jaundice is commonly produced by therapeutic doses of:

(A) mesterolone
(B) methyltestosterone
(C) nandrolone
(D) testosterone

429 The uterus of the immature rat responds by hypertrophy and hyperplasia to a hormonal product of the ovarian follicle. Which of the following synthetic steroids will produce a similar uterotrophic action?

(A) norgestrel
(B) mestranol
(C) mesterolone
(D) cyproterone

Type 2

Which substance best fits each description?

430 the active androgen at most target tissues
431 an androgen with a preponderance of anabolic actions
432 used orally in the treatment of menopausal symptoms
433 a progestogen used in oral contraceptive tablets

Options for 430–433:

(A)   ethinyloestradiol
(B)   progesterone
(C)   fluoxymesterone
(D)   17β-oestradiol
(E)   norethandrolone
(F)   5α-dihydrotestosterone
(G)   norethisterone

For each drug select the option which best describes its action.

434   stilboestrol [diethylstilbestrol]
435   norethynodrel
436   clomiphene
437   cyproterone

Options for 434–437:

(A)   an agonist at androgen receptors
(B)   an antagonist at androgen receptors
(C)   an agonist at oestrogen receptors
(D)   an antagonist at oestrogen receptors
(E)   an agonist at progestogen receptors
(F)   an antagonist at progestogen receptors

A group of adult animals has been ovariectomised (ovaries surgically removed). How would the following responses be affected by this operation?

438   uterine weight increase produced by 17β-oestradiol
439   uterine weight increase produced by follicle-stimulating hormone
440   the increase in serum gonadotrophin secretion produced by clomiphene

Options for 438–440:

(A)   operation increases response
(B)   operation does not consistently affect the response
(C)   operation reduces response

A group of male rats has been given a single injection of α-chlorhydrin. How would the following measurements be influenced by the pretreatment?

441 their sexual activity 1 week after injection B
442 their sexual activity 10 weeks after injection B
443 their fertility 1 week after injection C
444 their fertility 10 weeks after injection B

Options for 441–444:

(A) pretreatment increases response
(B) pretreatment hardly affects response
(C) pretreatment reduces response

The following drugs act indirectly by altering the secretion of an endogenous hormone. For each drug and effect select the appropriate hormone.

445 ethanol prevention of milk ejection
446 prostaglandin $F_{2\alpha}$ abortifacient action early in pregnancy
447 stilboestrol [diethylstilbestrol] used to treat prostatic carcinoma
448 bromocriptine used to treat female infertility

Options for 445–448:

(A) 17β-oestradiol
(B) progesterone
(C) testosterone
(D) antidiuretic hormone
(E) oxytocin
(F) prolactin
(G) human chorionic gonadotrophin

During early puberty, which drugs or radiations would be expected to produce the following effects?

449 increased sperm count and seminal vesicle weight
450 decreased sperm count but with little effect on seminal vesicle weight
451 decreased sperm count and increased seminal vesicle weight
452 decreased sperm count and seminal vesicle weight

Options for 449–452:

(A) corticosteroid
(B) androgen
(C) x-ray radiation

    (D)   follicle-stimulating hormone + luteinising hormone
    (E)   oestrogen

What stages of sperm production in the human are being stopped by the single doses of the drugs administered in *Figure 7*:

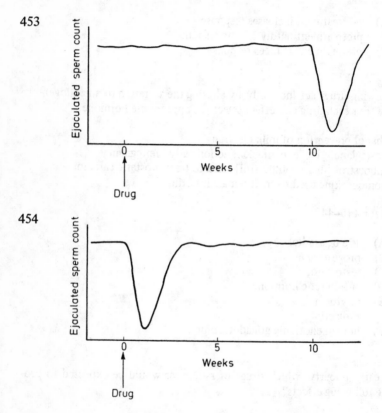

453

454

Figure 7

Options for 453–454:

    (A)   spermatids
    (B)   spermaceti
    (C)   spermatocytes
    (D)   Sertoli cells
    (E)   spermatozoa
    (F)   spermatogonia

How would the following actions of oestrogens be affected by concurrent administration of a progestogen?

455 contraceptive action
456 secretion by the uterine endometrium
457 thrombogenic action
458 intermenstrual bleeding
459 sperm penetration through cervical mucus
460 growth of ducts of mammary glands

Options for 455–460:

The action would be:

    (A) increased
    (B) hardly affected
    (C) decreased

Which of the steroid groups can be used for the treatment of:

461 benign prostatic hyperplasia
462 premenopausal inoperable carcinoma of the breast
463 prostatic carcinoma
464 inoperable carcinoma of the body of the uterus

Options for 461–464:

    (A) oestrogen
    (B) androgen
    (C) progestogen

Select the drug which:

465 has almost exclusively myometrial stimulant properties
466 has myometrial stimulant and luteolytic properties
467 has myometrial stimulant and slight vasoconstrictor properties
468 has pronounced vasoconstrictor and slight myometrial stimulant properties

Options for 465–468:

    (A) ergometrine
    (B) ergotamine
    (C) oxytocin
    (D) prostaglandin $F_{2\alpha}$

Which agents, administered to the mother during pregnancy, can produce in the offspring:

469   virilisation of the female fetus
470   phocomelia (absence of long bones)
471   cretinism
472   growth retardation but not cleft palate
473   vaginal adenocarcinoma

Options for 469–473:

(A)   carbimazole
(B)   oestradiol
(C)   stilboestrol [diethylstilbestrol]
(D)   testosterone
(E)   thalidomide
(F)   tobacco smoking

In women taking the oestrogen plus progestogen oral contraceptive, compared with controls, the incidence of:

474   ovulation
475   benign breast neoplasms
476   cerebrovascular disease
477   irregular cycle length
478   diabetes

Options for 474–478:

(A)   is higher
(B)   is about the same
(C)   is lower

Most groups of hormones are defined by their biological actions which have become the basis of biological assay systems. Which drug would you expect to be active in the following test systems?

479   The Allen Doisy assay which estimates the degree of cornification of the vaginal epithelium in the rat
480   Clauberg's test in which the transformation of a proliferative endometrium to a secretory endometrium in the rabbit is observed

481 The assay system which is based on the increase in size of the cock's comb first observed to be hormonally dependent by Berthold

482 The Ashheim and Zondek test system in which the biological response is the increase in ovarian weight of immature mice

Options for 479–482:

    (A) stilboestrol [diethylstilbestrol]
    (B) human chorionic gonadotrophin
    (C) norgestrel
    (D) testosterone propionate

Type 4

483 induces progesterone synthesis by the corpus luteum
484 promotes luteolysis
485 induces uterine contractions only at term
486 can cause a teratogenic effect in the first and second trimesters of pregnancy
487 blocks the synthesis of prostaglandins *in vivo*

Options for 483–487:

    (A) indomethacin
    (B) methotrexate
    (C) oxytocin
    (D) luteinising hormone
    (E) prostaglandin $F_{2\alpha}$

488 sexual immaturity, short stature, amenorrhoea, 'webbing' of the neck and, later, osteoporosis
489 increased secretion of androgens, treated with corticosteroids
490 decreased secretion of oestrogens and progesterone with increased androgen secretion by the ovary
491 presence of both testicular and ovarian tissue

Options for 488–491:

    (A) true hermaphroditism
    (B) female Turner's syndrome
    (C) Klinefelter's syndrome
    (D) adrenogenital syndrome
    (E) polycystic ovarian (Stein–Leventhal) syndrome

Type 5

During the first half of the menstrual cycle, or (492) phase, the blood contains a relatively high concentration of (493) derived from the (494). Secretion of (493) can be inhibited by (495) which acts at the (496). (497) secretion by the thecal cells of the ovary leads to proliferation of the uterine endometrium. At midcycle (498) produces ovulation and also induces the formation of a corpus luteum which secretes (499). (499) produces a (500) uterine endometrium during the second half of the cycle.

Options for 492–500:

492   (A)   epididymal
      (B)   luteal
      (C)   follicular
      (D)   tubular

493   (A)   follicle-stimulating hormone
      (B)   human chorionic gonadotrophin
      (C)   luteinising hormone
      (D)   prolactin

494   (A)   hypothalamus
      (B)   anterior pituitary gland
      (C)   ovary
      (D)   uterus

495   (A)   clomiphene
      (B)   ethinyloestradiol
      (C)   dexamethasone
      (D)   triiodothyronine

496   (A)   hypothalamus
      (B)   posterior pituitary gland
      (C)   ovary
      (D)   uterus

497   (A)   oestriol
      (B)   prostaglandin E_2
      (C)   progesterone
      (D) 17β-oestradiol

498   (A)   follicle-stimulating hormone
      (B)   human chorionic gonadotrophin

    (C)   luteinising hormone
    (D)   prolactin

499 (A)   oestriol
      (B) 17β-oestradiol
      (C)   prostaglandin E_2
      (D)   progesterone

500 (A)   proliferative
      (B)   secretory
      (C)   cornified
      (D)   haemorrhagic

The combined type of oral contraceptive tablet contains an oestrogen and a progestogen. Norethisterone and (501) are widely used progestogens. They are known as (502). Two oestrogens have been commonly used in combination with the progestogens; they are ethinyloestradiol and (503). It is recommended that not more than (504) of the oestrogen be incorporated into each tablet because of the slight risk of precipitating (505). The main site of action of the combined type of oral contraceptive tablet is thought to be at the (506) which results in suppression of (507). In contrast to this there are oral contraceptive preparations which consist only of progestogen. One of their major sites of action is believed to be on the (508) which results in alteration of (509). These latter preparations are (510) the combined type tablet and if fertilisation occurs there is a higher incidence of (511).

Options for 501–511:

501 (A)   norethandrolone
      (B)   norgestrel
      (C)   mestranol
      (D)   nandrolone

502 (A)   17-OH progestogens
      (B)   17-oxosteroids
      (C)   19-norsteroids
      (D) C_{19} compounds

503 (A)   chlorotrianisene
      (B)   quinestrol
      (C)   mestranol
      (D)   stilboestrol [diethylstilbestrol]

504 (A) 50 mg
     (B) 30 µg
     (C) 50 µg
     (D) 100 µg

505 (A) thromboembolism
     (B) amenorrhoea
     (C) hypertension
     (D) cardiac failure

506 (A) hypothalamus-pituitary gland
     (B) oviduct
     (C) ovary
     (D) cervix

507 (A) oviductal motility
     (B) sperm penetration into the uterus
     (C) ovulation
     (D) uterine motility

508 (A) hypothalamus-pituitary gland
     (B) vagina
     (C) ovary
     (D) cervix

509 (A) vaginal pH
     (B) sperm penetration into the uterus
     (C) ovulation
     (D) progesterone secretion

510 (A) more effective than
     (B) less effective than
     (C) as effective as

511 (A) thromboembolism
     (B) ectopic pregnancy
     (C) abortion
     (D) uterine bleeding

(512) is a protein hormone secreted by the (513) which initiates and maintains (514). During pregnancy, proliferation of the lobuloalveolar system of
the (515) is produced by this hormone in combination with the ovarian steroid secretions, (516), and other hormonal support. Postpartum, successful

fant feeding is also dependent upon the release of (517) from the (518)
contracting the smooth muscle of the (519). (514) may be undesirable
nd can be suppressed by high doses of (520). The use of these drugs is
ssociated with serious side-effects to the mother, e.g. (521), and conse-
uently they have been replaced with the dopaminergic drug, (522).

ptions for 512–522:

12 **(A)** oxytocin
   (B) luteinising hormone
   (C) prolactin
   (D) vasopressin

13 **(A)** anterior pituitary gland
   (B) posterior pituitary gland
   (C) hypothalamus
   (D) pineal gland

514 **(A)** fetal growth
    (B) fertility
    (C) pregnancy
    (D) lactation

515 **(A)** uterus
    (B) placenta
    (C) mammary gland
    (D) fetal lung

516 **(A)** 17β-oestradiol and progesterone
    (B) oestriol and dihydrotestosterone
    (C) androstenedione and aldosterone
    (D) oestrone and pregnanediol

517 **(A)** oxytocin
    (B) luteinising hormone
    (C) prolactin
    (D) vasopressin

518 **(A)** anterior pituitary gland
    (B) posterior pituitary gland
    (C) hypothalamus
    (D) pineal gland

519 (A) myometrium
     (B) mammary arterial endothelium
     (C) mammary ducts
     (D) mammary alveoli

520 (A) oestrogens
     (B) mineralocorticoids
     (C) glucocorticoids
     (D) phenothiazines

521 (A) hirsutism (excessive hair growth)
     (B) menorrhagia (excessive menstrual bleeding)
     (C) thromboembolism
     (D) anaemia

522 (A) bromocriptine
     (B) apomorphine
     (C) tyramine
     (D) ergotamine

The mean age at which the menopause occurs is (523) years. The gradu
senescence of the (524) leads to a decline in the plasma concentrations
sex steroids and consequent bodily changes. Hormonal replacement therap
will reverse many of the bodily changes but not (525); however, breal
through bleeding is a common side-effect when (526) therapy is used.

Options for 523–526:

523 (A) 55
     (B) 50
     (C) 45
     (D) 40

524 (A) adrenal gland
     (B) ovary
     (C) anterior pituitary gland
     (D) hypothalamus

525 (A) senile vaginitis
     (B) vasomotor changes
     (C) osteoporosis
     (D) depression

526 (A) intermittent oestrogen plus progestogen
(B) intermittent oestrogen plus androgen
(C) continuous oestrogen
(D) continuous progestogen

The differentiation of cells in the embryonic gonads to form oögonia or spermatogonia can be influenced (527). Formation of oöcytes occurs (528). Development of sperm beyond spermatogonia takes place (529). In the genetic male Wolffian duct development can be prevented by (530). Wolffian ducts will grow in genetic females given (531).

Options for 527–531:

527 (A) by androgens
(B) by androgen antagonists
(C) by progestogens
(D) only by the genetic composition of the embryo

528 (A) well before birth
and (B) near the time of birth
529 (C) between birth and puberty
(D) during and after puberty

530 (A) cyproterone acetate
and (B) ethinyloestradiol
531 (C) medroxyprogesterone acetate
(D) testosterone propionate

$A = X > Y$
$B = X = Y$
$C = Y > X$

Type 6

532 (X) the follicle-stimulating hormone concentration in plasma during most of the menstrual cycle
(Y) the follicle-stimulating hormone concentration in plasma soon after the menopause

533 (X) the contraceptive efficiency of intrauterine contraceptive devices
(Y) the contraceptive efficiency of the sequential type of oral contraceptive

534 (X) the anabolic action of 17β-oestradiol
(Y) the anabolic action of testosterone

535 (X)   total prostaglandin concentration in human semen
     (Y)   total prostaglandin concentration in human blood

536 (X)   the time to onset of sterility produced by a male contraceptive
           which acts upon epididymal sperm
     (Y)   the time to onset of sterility produced by a male contraceptive
           which acts upon spermatogonial division

537 (X)   the duration of action of testosterone
     (Y)   the duration of action of testosterone propionate

538 (X)   sperm penetration of cervical mucus during the use of the proges-
           togen-only type of oral contraceptive
     (Y)   sperm penetration of cervical mucus during the use of the com-
           bined type of oral contraceptive

539 (X)   the contraceptive efficiency of the progestogen-only type of oral
           contraceptive
     (Y)   the contraceptive efficiency of the combined type of oral contra-
           ceptive

540 (X)   the ratio of myotropic to androgenic activity of testosterone
     (Y)   the ratio of myotropic to androgenic activity of norethandrolone

541 (X)   the ratio of myotropic to androgenic activity of fluoxymesterone
     (Y)   the ratio of myotropic to androgenic activity of norandrolone

542 (X)   the androgenic potency of 5α-dihydrotestosterone
     (Y)   the androgenic potency of testosterone

543 (X)   the androgenic potency of androsterone
     (Y)   the androgenic potency of 5α-dihydrotestosterone

544 (X)   the rate of metabolism of barbiturates in men
     (Y)   the rate of metabolism of barbiturates in women

545 In women aged 20–25:
     (X)   the death rate associated with the use of an inefficient means of
           contraception and any consequent pregnancies
     (Y)   the death rate associated with the use of the combined type of
           oral contraceptive and any consequent pregnancies

546 In women aged 40–45:
     (X)   the death rate associated with the use of an inefficient means of
           contraception and any consequent pregnancies

QMUL Library

Borrowed Items 22/11/2010 23:09
XXXXXXX3421

Item Title	Due Date
Medical biochemistry	29/11/2010
An introduction to dental ma	29/11/2010
The anatomical basis of den	24/11/2010
Netter's head and neck anat	24/11/2010
Anatomy and physiology : fr	25/11/2010
* Pharmacology	20/12/2010
* 1200 multiple choice quest	29/11/2010

* Indicates items borrowed today
Thank you for using this unit

(Y) the death rate associated with the use of the combined type of oral contraceptives and any consequent pregnancies

47 The pregnancy rate in women in the 6 months after discontinuing contraception by means of:
(X) an intrauterine device
(Y) the combined oestrogen and progestogen tablet

548 The incidence of nausea and vomiting when prostaglandins are used:
(X) to terminate pregnancy during the second trimester
(Y) to induce labour at term

549 The incidence of death associated with taking the combined type of oral contraceptive in women aged:
(X) 20–25 years
(Y) 35–40 years

550 (X) the frequency of ovulation during oral contraception with ethinyl-oestradiol and norethisterone
(Y) the frequency of ovulation during oral contraception with northisterone

551 (X) the dose of oestrogen required for the suppression of lactation
(Y) the dose of oestrogen required for the suppression of ovulation

552 (X) the dose of oestrogen required for the suppression of ovulation
(Y) the dose of oestrogen required for the treatment of inoperable carcinoma of the breast

Type 8

553 Prostaglandin $F_{2\alpha}$ can produce abortion in early pregnancy in animals

BECAUSE

prostaglandin $F_{2\alpha}$ is luteolytic

554 Norethisterone cannot be taken safely during pregnancy

BECAUSE

norethisterone possesses significant androgenic potency

555   Cyclophosphamide will produce sterility in males

BECAUSE

cyclophosphamide is an alkylating agent

556   Mesterolone will increase the rate of spermatogenesis

BECAUSE

mesterolone is an androgen

557   High doses of oestrogens given within 3 days after coitus are contraceptive

BECAUSE

oestrogens decrease anterior pituitary secretion of the gonadotrophins

558   Thalidomide produced its major teratogenic effect when administered around day 100 of human pregnancy

BECAUSE

the period of organogenesis occurs around day 100 of human pregnancy

559   Cyproterone acetate is used to prevent the effects of excess androgen secretion

BECAUSE

cyproterone acetate competes with androgens for their receptors

560   Acne vulgaris can be treated by administration of 19-nortestosterone derivatives

BECAUSE

acne vulgaris results from underproduction of androgens

561 The mortality rate is greater than the expected
sum of the contributions of the individual risk
factors in women who smoke cigarettes and also
use oral contraceptives

BECAUSE

cigarette smoking increases the incidence of
malignant disease

562 Stilboestrol [diethylstilbestrol] is preferred to
ethinyloestradiol in conjunction with a progestogen
for treatment of Turner's syndrome

BECAUSE

ethinyloestradiol tends to cause deep pigmentation
of the nipples in these patients, which is cosmetically
undesirable

563 Drugs are most likely to produce teratogenic effects
on the fetus when administered to the mother
3–14 weeks after the last menstrual period

BECAUSE

3–14 weeks after the last menstrual period is the
time of organogenesis in humans

564 Intrauterine devices prevent implantation in the
oviduct

BECAUSE

intrauterine devices stop ovulation

565 Intrauterine devices can produce excessive
uterine bleeding

BECAUSE

intrauterine devices interfere with the
hypothalamic-pituitary control of the menstrual
cycle

566   Phenytoin [diphenyl-hydantoin] plus pheno-
      barbitone can increase the incidence of cleft lip
      and/or cleft palate

      BECAUSE

      phenytoin plus phenobarbitone has a significant
      action in inhibiting the formation of
      tetrahydrofolate

567   Mesterolone is used in preference to fluoxymesterone
      in the treatment of male hypogonadism

      BECAUSE

      mesterolone, whilst stimulating spermatogenesis,
      does not cause testicular atrophy

568   The tetracyclines are the first choice in the
      treatment of acne; however, in resistant
      cases in females, mesterolone can be used

      BECAUSE

      a major contributory factor to the
      continuation of acne in females is the cyclic
      ovarian production of androgens

569   Bromocriptine may be used for the treatment
      of acromegaly

      BECAUSE

      bromocriptine decreases the plasma concentration
      of prolactin

Type 9

570   The following mechanisms are responsible for the contraceptive action
      of the sequential type of oral contraceptives:

      (A)   inhibition of mid-cycle surge of luteinising hormone secretion
      (B)   inhibition of follicle-stimulating hormone secretion
      (C)   effect on endometrium
      (D)   rendering cervical mucus hostile to sperm

571   Spermatogenesis:

   (A)   requires follicle-stimulating hormone
   (B)   requires luteinising hormone
   (C)   is increased by high doses of testosterone propionate
   (D)   is decreased by 17β-oestradiol

572   After the menopause:

   (A)   plasma follicle-stimulating hormone concentrations are decreased
   (B)   plasma 17β-oestradiol concentrations are decreased
   (C)   ovarian responses to luteinising hormone are decreased
   (D)   ovarian responses to follicle-stimulating hormone are decreased

573   Nandrolone:

   (A)   increases seminal vesicle weight
   (B)   increases muscle growth
   (C)   promotes bone epiphyseal fusion
   (D)   promotes male fertility

574   Oxytocin:

   (A)   increases milk secretion
   (B)   is secreted in response to suckling
   (C)   secretion can be inhibited by ethanol
   (D)   is used to induce labour

575   Human chorionic gonadotrophin:

   (A)   is secreted by trophoblastic tissue
   (B)   increases ovarian progesterone secretion
   (C)   concentration in urine is measured to confirm pregnancy
   (D)   has actions most resembling follicle-stimulating hormone
   (E)   is used to promote fertility in women

576   Luteinising hormone/follicle-stimulating hormone-releasing hormone:

   (A)   is synthesised by neurones within the hypothalamus

(B)   is transported to the anterior pituitary gland via a portal blood supply

(C)   when injected will increase gonadotrophin secretion

(D)   is therapeutically useful in male and female infertility

(E)   is inactive orally

577   Synthesis of specific sex steroid hormone-binding protein by the liver is increased in patients being treated with:

(A)   stilboestrol [diethylstilbestrol]

(B)   clomiphene

(C)   oral contraceptives

(D)   metyrapone

578   In a female being treated with an oestrogen and a progestogen (for example, with the combined type of oral contraceptive):

(A)   stopping both the oestrogen and the progestogen will lead to withdrawal bleeding

(B)   stopping only the progestogen will lead to withdrawal bleeding

(C)   stopping only the oestrogen will lead to withdrawal bleeding

579   Testosterone derivatives are:

(A)   androgenic

(B)   anabolic

(C)   diabetogenic

(D)   progestogenic

(E)   carcinogenic (liver)

580   In the male, the pituitary secretion of the gonadotrophins can be decreased by:

(A)   clomiphene

(B) 17β-oestradiol

(C)   testosterone

(D) 5α-dihydrotestosterone

(E)   progesterone

81 The administration of testosterone to the prepubertal human male leads to:

(A) thickening of the vocal cords
(B) enlargement of the penis and scrotum
(C) general increase in subcutaneous fat
(D) closure of the epiphyses
(E) growth of axillary, facial and pubic hair

82 Male infertility is particularly resistant to treatment. However, the following drugs do, in certain circumstances, improve testicular function:

(A) mesterolone
(B) mestranol
(C) luteinising hormone/follicle-stimulating hormone-releasing hormone
(D) clomiphene
(E) human chorionic gonadotrophin

583 Hormone-dependent carcinomas of the mammary glands can be treated with:

(A) testosterone
(B) tamoxifen
(C) ethinyloestradiol
(D) cyclophosphamide

584 Clinical applications of the anabolic effects of androgenic steroids are in:

(A) debility
(B) anaemia
(C) oligospermia
(D) osteoporosis

585 Pituitary secretion of the gonadotrophins can be suppressed by:

(A) progesterone
(B) testosterone
(C) 5α-dihydrotestosterone
(D) 17β-oestradiol

   (E)   methallibure
   (F)   aldosterone

586   The adrenogenital syndrome in females can be due to enzyme defic
      iencies in the adrenal cortex leading to excess androgen secretion. The
      virilisation can be treated by giving:

   (A)   cyproterone
   (B)   ethinyloestradiol
   (C)   hydrocortisone

587   The oestrogen component of the combined type of oral contraceptive
      tablet may be responsible for the following unwanted effects seen in
      some women:

   (A)   cervical erosion
   (B)   hypertension
   (C)   acne
   (D)   thrombophlebitis
   (E)   pigmentation
   (F)   fluid retention

588   Testosterone, secreted by the fetal testis:

   (A)   prevents the development of the female reproductive tract
   (B)   causes the development of the male reproductive tract
   (C)   imprints the hypothalamus such that in adult life gonadotrophins
         are secreted in an acyclic manner

589   Prolactin secretion is:

   (A)   increased by bromocriptine
   (B)   increased by chlorpromazine
   (C)   increased by reserpine
   (D)   decreased by apomorphine

590   Testosterone in the female:

   (A)   induces hirsutism

(B)   produces nitrogen retention
(C)   does not alter plasma gonadotrophin concentrations
(D)   thickens the vocal cords

91   The release of prolactin from the anterior pituitary gland is:

(A)   stimulated by cutting the pituitary stalk
(B)   controlled by a release-inhibiting neurohumour
(C)   unaffected by the synthetic thyrotrophin-releasing factors
(D)   increased by the phenothiazine major tranquillizers

92   After the menopause the following changes occur in women:

(A)   osteoporosis
(B)   atrophy of the uterus
(C)   cessation of ovulation
(D)   decreased plasma oestrogen and progesterone concentrations
(E)   decreased plasma follicle-stimulating hormone and luteinising
      hormone concentrations

93   In a menopausal woman, the cyclical use of exogenous oestrogens will:

(A)   decrease the frequency of hot flushes
(B)   increase plasma follicle-stimulating hormone concentrations
(C)   be followed by withdrawal bleeding
(D)   increase the chance of developing uterine endometrial carcinoma

94   The following drugs have been used to suppress lactation:

(A)   stilboestrol [diethylstilbestrol]
(B)   chlorotrianisene
(C)   testosterone propionate
(D)   bromocriptine
(E)   clomiphene citrate

95   The following are examples of the use of hormones in replacement
     therapy:

(A)   thyroxine for myxoedema

    (B)   oestrogens for menopausal symptoms
    (C)   oestrogens plus progestogens for endometriosis (extrauterine growth of uterine endometrium)
    (D)   insulin for diabetes mellitus

596 19-nortesterone derivatives which possess progestogenic activity are particular useful alone or in combination with oestrogen for:

    (A)   fertility regulation
    (B)   dysmenorrhoea
    (C)   menopausal symptoms
    (D)   endometriosis
    (E)   habitual abortion

4 Central Nervous System Pharmacology

Type 1

597 Ferguson's principle is best described by:

(A) drugs acting by structurally non-specific mechanisms will produce quantitatively similar pharmacological actions when present in the biophase at equimolar concentrations

(B) the thermodynamic activities of drugs acting by structurally non-specific mechanisms are independent of phase when the phases are in equilibrium

(C) drugs acting by structurally non-specific mechanisms will produce the same quantitative effect at the same relative saturation of the biophase

(D) drugs acting by structurally non-specific mechanisms are depressants of biological activity

(E) there is a causal relationship between lipid solubility and the anaesthetic potency of general anaesthetics

598 The transmitter liberated from the α-motoneurone collateral at its synapse with the Renshaw cell is:

(A) noradrenaline [norepinephrine]
(B) acetylcholine
(C) dopamine
(D) glycine
(E) γ-aminobutyric acid (GABA)

599   Nalorphine is not used clinically as an analgesic because:

(A)   it is hallucinogenic
(B)   its analgesic activity is too weak
(C)   it is poorly absorbed from the gastrointestinal tract
(D)   it is emetic

600   A physician suspecting that a patient has become physically dependent on methadone prescribed postoperatively should:

(A)   change the medication to an antipyretic analgesic
(B)   change the medication to the non-addictive opiate pentazocine
(C)   reduce the daily dose of methadone gradually
(D)   continue with the dose schedule, since the subsequent withdrawal symptoms will be mild
(E)   terminate all medication

The following paragraph describes the course of drugs given during a short operation. The anaesthetist had a limited number of anaesthetics available.

The patient was premedicated with chlorpromazine and pentazocine. Anaesthesia was induced by inhalation of 10% ether and then maintained with 5% ether. Immediately after induction atropine was deemed necessary and an intravenous injection given. At this stage muscle relaxation was inadequate and an intravenous injection of tubocurarine was given. The operation was completed in 20 min and the anaesthetic was discontinued. Neostigmine was then injected. Over-enthusiastic postoperative administration of pentazocine required reversal and the drug of choice was given intravenously.
Use this information for questions 601–611.

601   Why was chlorpromazine given?

(A)   to preclude excessive cardiovascular depression
(B)   to minimise pentazocine-induced respiratory depression
(C)   to potentiate the analgesic action of pentazocine
(D)   to improve muscle relaxation
(E)   to allay anxiety and minimise the risk of vomiting

602   Immediately prior to induction of anaesthesia the patient's pupils would have been:

(A)   dilated
(B)   constricted
(C)   of normal size

03　If halothane had been used instead of ether, the rate of induction
　　would have been:

　　(A)　faster
　　(B)　slower
　　(C)　the same rate

504　Why was the atropine necessary?

　　(A)　to increase the heart rate following ether-induced cardiac depres-
　　　　sion
　　(B)　to reduce the heart rate following ether-induced cardiac stimula-
　　　　tion
　　(C)　to reduce exocrine secretions
　　(D)　to minimise pentazocine-induced respiratory depression

505　If halothane had been used as the anaesthetic the dose of tubocurarine
　　required would have been:

　　(A)　larger
　　(B)　smaller
　　(C)　the same

606　Why was the injection of neostigmine necessary?

　　(A)　to accelerate recovery from the anaesthetic
　　(B)　to reverse the action of atropine
　　(C)　to reverse the action of tubocurarine
　　(D)　to potentiate the action of pentazocine

607　Recovery from the anaesthetic action of ether was due to:

　　(A)　redistribution of the anaesthetic into other tissues
　　(B)　excretion of the unchanged drug from the lungs
　　(C)　acute tolerance
　　(D)　metabolism of the drug

608   What was the drug of choice for reversal of the action of pentazocine?

    (A)   methylamphetamine
    (B)   nikethamide
    (C)   nalorphine
    (D)   naloxone

609   In the likely (or unlikely) event of cardiac arrhythmias occurring, which one of the following drugs would not have been beneficial?

    (A)   cocaine
    (B)   lignocaine [lidocaine]
    (C)   phenytoin [diphenylhydantoin]
    (D)   procainamide
    (E)   propranolol

610   Would the combination of drugs used cause respiratory depression to the extent that artificial ventilation would be necessary?

    (A)   yes
    (B)   no

611   If cyclopropane had been used instead of ether, the likelihood of cardiac arrhythmias would have been

    (A)   greater
    (B)   smaller
    (C)   the same

Type 2

Figure 8 compares the agonist to antagonist ratios of narcotic analgesics. Position **A** represents a drug with almost pure agonist activity while position **E** represents a pure antagonist.
    Indicate the position of the following drugs:

612   levallorphan
613   levorphanol
614   nalorphine
615   naloxone
616   pentazocine

Options for 612–616:

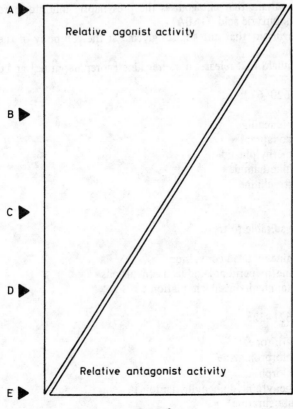

A ▶

Relative agonist activity

B ▶

C ▶

D ▶

Relative antagonist activity

E ▶

Figure 8

Many drug molecules are optically active. Which is the pharmacologically active isomer for:

617 the respiratory stimulant action of amphetamine
618 the cough suppressant activity of methorphan
619 the respiratory depressant action of hexobarbitone

Options for 617–619:

(A) due predominantly to the *l*-isomer
(B) due predominantly to the *d*-isomer
(C) not predominantly due to either optical isomer

Which substance best fits each description?

620   A convulsant that antagonises the presynaptic inhibitory transmitter γ-aminobutyric acid (GABA)

621   A convulsant that antagonises glycine at the cell body of the α-moto-neurone

622   A stimulant that releases noradrenaline [norepinephrine] and dopamine

Options for 620–622:

    (A)   bicuculline
    (B)   doxapram
    (C)   methylphenidate
    (D)   nikethamide
    (E)   strychnine

Select a drug suitable to treat:

623   strychnine-induced convulsions
624   pethidine [meperidine] -induced convulsions
625   amphetamine-induced stimulation

Options for 621–625:

    (A)   barbitone
    (B)   chlorpromazine
    (C)   nalorphine
    (D)   phenytoin [diphenylhydantoin]
    (E)   tubocurarine

Which substance best fits each description?

626   An analeptic which increases respiration by stimulating the reticular formation and carotid bodies

627   An orally effective sympathomimetic, with central stimulant activity which is used in the prophylaxis of asthma

628   A central stimulant that antagonises a neurotransmitter which has a presynaptic inhibitory action

629   A central stimulant and bronchodilator which increases the concentration of $3',5'$-cyclic AMP by inhibiting phosphodiesterase

630   A bronchodilator which is inactive orally and which increases the concentration of $3',5'$-cyclic AMP by a mechanism not involving inhibition of phosphodiesterase

Options for 626–630:

    (A)   adrenaline [epinephrine]
    (B)   caffeine
    (C)   doxapram
    (D)   ephedrine
    (E)   nikethamide
    (F)   picrotoxin

Drugs produce their effects on the central nervous system by a variety of mechanisms. After injection in an experimental animal:

631   amphetamine
632   atropine
633   chlorpromazine
634   eserine
635   haloperidol
636   hyoscine [scopolamine]
637   imipramine
638   phenelzine
639   pilocarpine
640   reserpine
641   methylphenidate

Options for 631–641:

    (A)   directly or indirectly activates central muscarinic receptors and causes hypothermia and tremor
    (B)   reduces activation of central muscarinic receptors and causes excitation
    (C)   reduces activation of central muscarinic receptors and causes sedation
    (D)   directly or indirectly activates central monoamine receptors and causes excitation and hyperthermia without prolongation of barbiturate-induced hypnosis
    (E)   directly or indirectly activates central monoamine receptors and causes excitation, hyperthermia and prolongation of barbiturate-induced hypnosis
    (F)   directly or indirectly activates central monoamine receptors and causes sedation without markedly affecting body temperature
    (G)   directly or indirectly reduces activation of central monoamine receptors and causes akinesia, sedation and hypothermia

For each of the following drugs select the appropriate description:

642 apomorphine
643 pholcodine
644 dextromethorphan
645 diamorphine (heroin)

Options for 642–645:

(A) a selective emetic devoid of analgesic activity
(B) a potent narcotic agonist well absorbed orally which has little sedative or euphoric action
(C) a pure narcotic antagonist devoid of narcotic agonist action
(D) a weak narcotic agonist which has a quantitatively selective action on the cough centre
(E) an effective cough suppressant which has no analgesic properties
(F) a potent narcotic agonist which causes considerable euphoria and sedation
(G) a narcotic antagonist analgesic in clinical use which does not produce morphine-like physical dependence

Figure 9 compares the agonist to antagonist ratios of narcotic analgesics. Position A represents a drug with almost pure agonist activity while position D represents a pure antagonist. Indicate the position of the following drugs:

646 buprenorphine
647 codeine
648 naloxone
649 pentazocine

Options for 646–649:

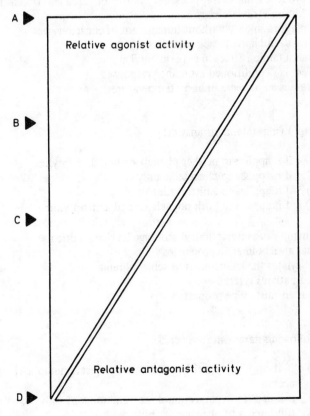

Figure 9

Type 3

For the following statements answer:

(A) if it applies to neither chlordiazepoxide nor chlorpromazine
(B) if it applies to chlordiazepoxide only
(C) if it applies to chlorpromazine only
(D) if it applies to both chlordiazepoxide and chlorpromazine

650 effectively reduces the hallucinosis induced by lysergic acid diethylamide
651 promotes relaxation of skeletal muscle
652 has antidepressant properties

653   its sedating effects are increased by alcohol
654   it produces an extrapyramidal motor disturbance which resembles Parkinson's disease
655   it reduces anxiety without impairment of consciousness
656   it has useful antiemetic properties
657   it has a taming effect in experimental animals
658   it reduces conditioned avoidance responses
659   it causes an increase in body temperature

For the following statements answer:

(A)   if it applies to neither phenelzine nor amitriptyline
(B)   if it applies to phenelzine only
(C)   if it applies to amitriptyline only
(D)   if it applies to both phenelzine and amitriptyline

660   its many drug interactions discourage its therapeutic use
661   it has anticholinergic properties
662   it alleviates the hallucinosis of schizophrenia
663   it potentiates tyramine
664   it has antihistamine properties

For the following statements answer:

(A)   if it applied to neither paracetamol [acetaminophen] nor phenacetin
(B)   if it applies to paracetamol [acetaminophen] only
(C)   if it applies to phenacetin only
(D)   if it applies to both paracetamol [acetaminophen] and phenacetin

665   antipyretic in analgesic doses
666   causes gastric bleeding
667   high doses produce methaemoglobinaemia
668   analgesic doses cause acid–base disturbance
669   high doses for prolonged periods carry the risk of renal damage

Type 4

670   imipramine
671   lithium
672   reserpine

73   phenelzine
74   amphetamine

ptions for 670–674:

(A)   depletes stored noradrenaline [norepinephrine]
(B)   inhibits noradrenaline [norepinephrine] re-uptake into nerves
(C)   blocks stimulated noradrenaline [norepinephrine] release without
      depleting noradrenaline [norepinephrine] stores
(D)   stoichiometrically releases noradrenaline [norepinephrine]
(E)   decreases production of acid metabolites from amine precursors

ndicate the mechanism of vomiting caused by:

75   apomorphine
76   cyclophosphamide
77   digoxin
78   disulphiram
79   metronidazole

Options for 675–679:

(A)   gastric irritation
(B)   labyrinthine stimulation
(C)   inhibiting aldehyde dehydrogenase
(D)   stimulating the chemoceptor trigger zone
(E)   stimulating the vomiting centre

580   acetylcholine
581   dopamine
582   glycine
683   5-hydroxytryptamine
684   prostaglandins

Options for 680–684:

(A)   an inhibitory transmitter in the striatum
(B)   synthesis inhibited by aspirin
(C)   specific depletion by *p*-chlorophenylalanine causes altered sleep
      pattern
(D)   inhibitory transmitter liberated from the Renshaw cell
(E)   liberated from motoneurone collateral

In rodents:

685   decrease locomotor activity, suppress conditioned avoidance respons and reverse reserpine hypothermia

686   decrease locomotor activity, suppress conditioned avoidance respons and cause ataxia and catatonia

687   decrease locomotor activity, suppress conditioned avoidance respons and cause ataxia and muscle relaxation

688   increase locomotor activity and reverse reserpine hypothermia

Options for 685–688:

(A)   benzodiazepine anxiolytics
(B)   centrally-acting sympathomimetics
(C)   phenothiazine neuroleptics
(D)   tricyclic antidepressants

689   A monoamine oxidase inhibitor which reverses established reserpir sedation

690   A monoamine oxidase inhibitor which does not reverse establishe reserpine sedation

691   A tricyclic antidepressant with relatively prominent sedative properties

692   The drug of choice in nocturnal enuresis

693   An amitriptyline-like antidepressant which has a marked stimulan action

694   An antidepressant related to benzodiazepine tranquillisers

695   A tranquilliser related to pethidine [meperidine]

696   An indole derivative which is a neuroleptic

697   An indole derivative which is a thymoleptic

Options for 689–697:

(A)   protriptyline
(B)   trimipramine
(C)   dibenzepine
(D)   amitriptyline
(E)   tranylcypromine
(F)   phenelzine
(G)   iprindole
(H)   haloperidol
(I)   oxypertine

Type 5

A 25-year-old male patient is admitted to hospital with a syndrome of retreat from reality, delusions, auditory hallucinations and bizarre regressive behaviour. He does not have tremor, high blood pressure or piloerection and there is no sign of excessive sweating. At first, chronic drug intoxication is suspected and (698) is thought to be most likely. When this has been excluded by urine analysis, (699) is diagnosed. Treatment with (700) is instituted and the patient improves. This drug (700) is believed to exert its effect by blocking (701) and as a consequence of this action, after 6 weeks of therapy new symptoms appear which include (702). Rather than withdraw the drug (700) a second drug (703) is prescribed which reduces the undesirable consequences of the first drug (700), but unfortunately the patient complains of (704). As a consequence (703) is withdrawn and the dosage of (700) is reduced.

Options for 698–704:

698 (A) LSD abuse
    (B) alcoholism
    (C) amphetamine abuse
    (D) cannabis abuse
    (E) narcotic withdrawal

699 (A) anxiety
    (B) endogenous depression
    (C) mania
    (D) psychomotor epilepsy
    (E) schizophrenia

700 (A) chlordiazepoxide
    (B) haloperidol
    (C) imipramine
    (D) phenelzine
    (E) phenytoin [diphenylhydantoin]

701 (A) β-adrenoceptors
    (B) muscarinic receptors
    (C) monoamine oxidase
    (D) receptors for dopamine
    (E) non-specifically, transmission at synapses within the central nervous system

702 (A) drowsiness
    (B) hypertension

    (C)   increased sensitivity to dietary amines
    (D)   hyperplasia of the gums
    (E)   rigidity and tremor

703 (A)   benztropine
    (B)   ephedrine
    (C)   phentolamine
    (D)   propranolol
    (E)   pilocarpine

704 (A)   blurred vision
    (B)   excessive salivation
    (C)   nausea
    (D)   tinnitus
    (E)   slow pulse

Type 6

705 (X)   the respiratory depressant action of pentobarbitone
    (Y)   the respiratory depressant action of a mixture of pentobarbitone and nalorphine

706 (X)   the respiratory depressant action of pentobarbitone
    (Y)   the respiratory depressant action of a mixture of pentobarbitone and naloxone

707 (X)   the speed of induction of anaesthesia with ether
    (Y)   the speed of induction of anaesthesia with a mixture of ether and 5% carbon dioxide

708 (X)   the antitussive action of diamorphine (heroin)
    (Y)   the antitussive action of an equianalgesic dose of morphine

709 (X)   the cardiovascular actions of amphetamine
    (Y)   the cardiovascular action of a dose of methylamphetamine equiactive as a central stimulant

710 (X)   the antiemetic action of chlorpromazine in the treatment of motion sickness
    (Y)   the antiemetic action of chlorpromazine in the treatment of vomiting in pregnancy

Type 8

711 Patients taking monoamine oxidase inhibitors
should avoid eating cheese

BECAUSE

cheese contains tyramine which is potentiated
by inhibition of liver monoamine oxidase thereby
causing a hypertensive crisis

712 Chlorpromazine enhances the hypnotic effect
of pentobarbitone

BECAUSE

chlorpromazine is a potent inhibitor of liver
oxidative enzymes

713 Urinary excretion of 5-hydroxyindole acetic acid
increases during the first day of reserpine therapy
in man

BECAUSE

reserpine releases 5-hydroxytryptamine from
tissue stores

714 Ethanol has a stimulant action on the brain
reticular activating system

BECAUSE

ethanol causes a selective increase in the oxygen
consumption of the brain reticular activating
system

715 Halogen-substituted anaesthetics can produce
cardiac arrhythmias

BECAUSE

halogen-substituted general anaesthetics can
sensitise the myocardium to the actions of
catecholamines

716   30% nitrous oxide causes analgesia

BECAUSE

30% nitrous oxide causes anaesthesia

717   Tetanus toxin causes spasm of skeletal muscle

BECAUSE

tetanus toxin prevents the release of inhibitory transmitter substance from the Renshaw cell at its synapse with the cell body of the α-motoneurone

718   Dopamine is effective in the treatment of Parkinson's disease after oral administration

BECAUSE

in Parkinson's disease there is a lack of dopamine in the corpus striatum

719   Monoamine oxidase inhibitors are frequently administered along with levodopa in the treatment of Parkinson's disease

BECAUSE

monoamine oxidase inhibitors inhibit L-dopa-decarboxylase in the periphery, thus reducing the rate of metabolism of levodopa

720   The phenothiazines (e.g. chlorpromazine) control sham rage in decorticate animals

BECAUSE

phenothiazines interfere with chemical neuro-transmission processes in the hypothalamus

721   Morphine reduces production of urine

BECAUSE

morphine causes release of antidiuretic hormone from the posterior pituitary gland

722   Dextromethorphan is a cough suppressant without
analgesic activity

BECAUSE

dextromethorphan is a *d*-isomer and the *d*-isomers
of the narcotic analgesics are selective cough
suppressants

723   1% halothane causes analgesia

BECAUSE

1% halothane causes anaesthesia

724   Nalorphine will antagonise the miotic action of
morphine

BECAUSE

nalorphine will antagonise all the excitatory
actions of morphine

725   Nalophine will not antagonise the respiratory
depressant action of pentazocine

BECAUSE

nalorphine is both a potent narcotic agonist
and antagonist

726   The tricyclic antidepressants have been used
to treat nocturnal enuresis in children

BECAUSE

tricyclic antidepressants have atropine-like effects

727   Monoamine oxidase inhibitors increase the
sedation due to reserpine

BECAUSE

monoamine oxidase inhibitors prevent the
intraneuronal metabolism of neurotransmitter
amines in the central nervous system

728   Phenothiazines (e.g. chlorpromazine) induce an extrapyramidal motor disturbance which resembles Parkinson's disease when administered for a long time

BECAUSE

phenothiazines block receptors for dopamine in the corpus striatum

729   Aspirin reduces the raised body temperature in man associated with excessive physical exercise

BECAUSE

aspirin acts as if to reset a hypothalamic thermostat

730   Levodopa is effective in the management of Parkinson's disease

BECAUSE

levodopa can raise the dopamine concentration in the corpus striatum in Parkinson's disease

Type 9

731   Morphine is a stereoanalogue of:

(A)   β-endorphin
(B)   des-tyr-γ-endorphin
(C)   leu-enkephalin
(D)   met-enkephalin
(E)   pethidine [meperidine]

732   Barbiturates:

(A)   possess local anaesthetic activity at high concentrations
(B)   will not interfere with the incidence of paradoxical (REM) sleep
(C)   will depress cellular oxidative enzymes
(D)   will induce liver microsomal enzymes
(E)   induce respiratory depression which is enhanced by nalorphine

733   Phenytoin [diphenylhydantoin] :

(A)   is effective in the treatment of some cardiac arrhythmias
(B)   causes relatively less depression of the medulla oblongata than equivalent anticonvulsant doses of phenobarbitone
(C)   can cause hyperplasia of the gums
(D)   increases post-tetanic potentiation originating from a cerebral ectopic focus
(E)   is useful in the treatment of grand mal epilepsy

734   Aspirin in a therapeutic dose:

(A)   causes sweating by a direct action on postganglionic nerves
(B)   acts in fever to reset the central thermostat
(C)   will not antagonise the hyperthermia of exercise
(D)   will cause more gastric bleeding than will equianalgesic doses of paracetamol [acetaminophen]

735   Phenylbutazone:

(A)   is as effective as aspirin as an antipyretic agent
(B)   causes agranulocytosis
(C)   causes gastric haemorrhage
(D)   is an anti-inflammatory agent
(E)   is more potent than aspirin as a uricosuric agent

736   Butyrophenones (e.g. haloperidol):

(A)   suppress the phenomenon of 'sham rage' in cats
(B)   are effective antipsychotic agents
(C)   are effective in the treatment of endogenous depression
(D)   cause extrapyramidal signs such as akinesia and tremor
(E)   may be used in neuroleptanalgesia

737   Halothane:

(A)   is a liquid at normal temperature and pressure
(B)   maintains anaesthesia at an inspired concentration of 1%
(C)   lacks selective skeletal muscle relaxant activity
(D)   sensitises the myocardium to catecholamines
(E)   is analgesic at subanaesthetic concentrations

738 Lysergic acid diethylamide:

    (A)   disrupts conditioned behaviour responses in mice
    (B)   induces cross-tolerance to mescaline
    (C)   induces hallucinosis which may be counteracted by phenothiazines
    (D)   induces hallucinosis which may be counteracted by imipramine
    (E)   produces marked effects on the autonomic nervous system mediated by its central action

739 The hazards of induction of anaesthesia by injection of thiopentone are:

    (A)   severe hypotension
    (B)   cessation of respiration
    (C)   necrosis following extravascular injection
    (D)   bronchospasm
    (E)   stimulation of bronchial and salivary secretion

740 Diazepam:

    (A)   is only mildly sedative at anxiolytic doses
    (B)   depresses spontaneous motor activity
    (C)   is a weak sympatholytic agent
    (D)   is antidepressant
    (E)   has a taming effect on aggressive animals

741 The stage of surgical anaesthesia is characterised by:

    (A)   electroencephalographic δ-waves and superimposed spindling
    (B)   an absence of autonomic and respiratory responses to pain
    (C)   miosis, diaphragmatic respiration and absence of laryngeal and pharyngeal reflexes
    (D)   absence of eye movements, normal pupil size, diaphragmatic respiration and decreased muscle tone

742 The phenothiazines (e.g. chlorpromazine):

    (A)   have antiemetic actions
    (B)   reduce aggression and defensive hostility in animals
    (C)   do not reduce vigilance and attention in man
    (D)   inhibit conditioned avoidance responses
    (E)   cause an extrapyramidal motor disturbance which resembles Parkinson's disease

743 The anticholinergic hallucinogens:

   (A)   disrupt conditioned avoidance and learned responses
   (B)   produce visual hallucinations
   (C)   cause mydriasis
   (D)   increase appetite
   (E)   cause an increase in heart rate

744 Phenacetin:

   (A)   is metabolised to paracetamol [acetaminophen] in the body
   (B)   is not antipyretic in analgesic doses
   (C)   causes methaemoglobinaemia
   (D)   is similar in analgesic potency to aspirin
   (E)   causes renal damage

745 Sodium valproate:

   (A)   is effective in grand mal epilepsy
   (B)   is effective in petit mal epilepsy
   (C)   can potentiate concurrently administered phenobarbitone
   (D)   should not be prescribed to children
   (E)   increases brain concentrations of γ-aminobutyric acid

746 Diazepam:

   (A)   does not cause physical dependence (addiction)
   (B)   causes amnesia
   (C)   is effective in status epilepticus
   (D)   is ineffective in schizophrenia

747 Signs of acute barbiturate poisoning include:

   (A)   opisthotonus (spasm of skeletal muscle)
   (B)   regular, shallow, infrequent breathing
   (C)   barely perceptible pulse
   (D)   dilated pupils
   (E)   coma

748   Dexamphetamine:

(A)   produces a decreased sense of fatigue
(B)   is used in the treatment of narcolepsy
(C)   produces an increase in appetite
(D)   when administered repeatedly induces tolerance

749   Imipramine:

(A)   causes euphoria in normal human volunteers
(B)   inhibits the action of acetylcholine at muscarinic receptors
(C)   is useful in the treatment of endogenous depression
(D)   enhances the effects of endogenous noradrenaline [norepinephrine]

750   Amylobarbitone:

(A)   induces tolerance
(B)   is a drug of physical dependence
(C)   is not analgesic at subanaesthetic doses
(D)   is a non-specific depressant of the central nervous system
(E)   has a higher lipid solubility than has thiopentone

751   Thiopentone:

(A)   is used to induce anaesthesia
(B)   is administered by intravenous injection
(C)   produces marked muscle relaxation
(D)   in low doses produces hyperalgesia

752   Phenobarbitone:

(A)   is used to treat grand mal epilepsy
(B)   may aggravate petit mal epilepsy
(C)   is slowly metabolised (compared to amylobarbitone)
(D)   produces skin rashes
(E)   has its effects terminated by tissue redistribution

753   Ethosuximide:

(A)   produces slight drowsiness in therapeutic doses
(B)   causes gastrointestinal disturbances
(C)   effectively suppresses absences due to petit mal epilspey
(D)   effectively suppresses absences due to temporal lobe epilepsy

54 β-lipotropin:

(A) is located in the pituitary gland
(B) is antagonised by naloxone
(C) has a shorter biological half-life than met-enkephalin
(D) is an analgesic
(E) is located in neurones in the limbic system

55 Both diazepam and thiopentone:

(A) have similar durations of action
(B) depress respiration
(C) induce tolerance
(D) cause dependence
(E) are suitable for intravenous injection
(F) cause amnesia

5 Human Antiparasitic Chemotherapy

including cancer chemotherapy

Type 1

756 A certain degree of selectivity exists within the alkylating group of cytotoxic drugs. Choose the malignant disease for which busulphan is the most appropriate chemotherapy:

(A) chronic lymphocytic leukaemia
(B) chronic myeloid leukaemia
(C) multiple myeloma

757 Select the class of antibiotic with the broadest spectrum of antimicrobial action:

(A) aminosugars (e.g. streptomycin)
(B) macrolides (e.g. erythromycin)
(C) penicillins
(D) tetracyclines

758 Sensitive bacteria are killed by the serum concentrations attained during clinical use of:

(A) chloramphenicol
(B) gentamicin
(C) sulphadimidine
(D) trimethoprim

Type 2

Select the most efficacious chemotherapy for:

759 hormone-dependent disseminated carcinoma of the breast in a young woman
760 disseminated carcinoma of the prostate
761 choriocarcinoma
762 polycythaemia vera
763 well-differentiated thyroid carcinoma
764 leukaemias
765 lymphomas

Options for 759–765:

(A) fluoxymesterone
(B) methotrexate
(C) radioactive gold
(D) radioactive iodide
(E) radioactive phosphorus (as phosphate)
(F) stilboestrol [diethylstilbestrol]

For each drug select the appropriate description:

766 chloramphenicol
767 isoniazid
768 lincomycin
769 streptomycin
770 sulphadimidine
771 tetracycline

Options for 766–771:

(A) penetrates bone well and is effective against Gram-positive bacteria including anaerobes (e.g. Bacteroides)
(B) is effective in tuberculosis but can cause generalised damage to peripheral nerves
(C) is ototoxic and effective in tuberculosis
(D) is a broad-spectrum antibiotic which may cause a fatal anaemia by stopping blood cell formation
(E) is the best treatment for a patient suffering from acute urinary tract infection for the first time
(F) is a broad-spectrum antibiotic which may cause discoloration of the teeth in children

For each drug select the appropriate description:

772   amphotericin
773   griseofulvin
774   nystatin
775   salicylic acid

Options for 772–775:

(A)   a topically applied keratolytic agent which eradicates tinea pedis ('athlete's foot')
(B)   a topically applied keratolytic agent which palliates tinea pedis
(C)   effective against *Candida albicans*, poorly absorbed from the gastrointestinal tract and not used to treat systemic infections
(D)   effective against *Candida albicans* and well absorbed from the gastrointestinal tract
(E)   effective against fungal nail infections and persists in the nails for weeks after oral administration
(F)   effective against fungal nail infections but does not persist in the nails for weeks after oral administration
(G)   effective against systemic mycoses, highly toxic and poorly absorbed from the gastrointestinal tract

Select the most appropriate treatment for each condition:

776   vaginal candidiasis
777   tinea of toe nails
778   tinea pedis not complicated by infection of the toe nails

Options for 776–778:

(A)   griseofulvin
(B)   nystatin
(C)   tolnaftate

Which drug best answers each of the following descriptions?

779   An inexpensive drug, very potent against Streptococci including pneumococci
780   A drug which is effective in infections with *Pseudomonas aeruginosa*
781   A relatively broad-spectrum antibiotic, well absorbed when administered by mouth

82   A drug which is useful in increasing the serum concentration of peni-
      cillin by decreasing tubular secretion

783 A drug active against penicillinase-producing Staphylococci

Options for 779–783:

    (A) amoxycillin
    (B) benzylpenicillin [penicillin G]
    (C) carbenicillin
    (D) cloxacillin
    (E) prednisolone
    (F) probenecid

Select the option which best describes how the cytotoxic effect of each agent
listed shows selectivity for the parasite cells rather than the host cells:

784   benzylpenicillin [penicillin G]
785   cephaloridine
786   chloramphenicol
787   cycloserine
788   dapsone (a sulphone)
789   erythromycin
790   methotrexate
791   nalidixic acid
792   nitrofurantoin
793   proguanil
794   pyrimethamine
795   rifampicin [rifampin]
796   sodium aminosalicylate
797   streptomycin
798   sulphadimidine
799   tetracycline
800   trimethoprim

Options for 784–800:

    (A) the drug interferes with a biochemical pathway in the parasite
         cell which is not present in the host cell
    (B) the drug interferes with a biochemical pathway which is common
         to both the parasite and host cells; however, in the parasite this
         pathway is more susceptible to the drug
    (C) the drug is accumulated by the parasite cells but not by the host
         cells

(D)   the drug is selectively distributed to a limited compartment of the host which forms the parasite's environment

Some chemotherapeutic agents owe their selectivity of action as normally used to two mechanisms which reinforce each other. One mechanism is selective administration or distribution of the drug to a limited compartment of the host which forms the parasite's environment. Select the reinforcing mechanism for each of the following:

801   bacitracin eyedrops
802   chloroquine tablets for malaria
803   griseofulvin tablets
804   idoxuridine eyedrops
805   malathion scalp application
806   neomycin eyedrops
807   nystatin pessaries
808   polymyxin eyedrops
809   quinine tablets for malaria
810   sulphacetamide eyedrops

Options for 801–810:

(A)   the drug interferes with a biochemical pathway in the parasite cell which is not present in the host cell
(B)   the drug interferes with a biochemical pathway which is common to host and parasite cells; however, in the parasite this pathway is more susceptible to the drug
(C)   the drug is selectively accumulated by the parasite

Choose the most appropriate option:

811   Prophylaxis against infective endocarditis with this drug is necessary in patients who have rheumatic valvular disease of the heart and who are undergoing dental extraction
812   Effective chemotherapy for the diarrhoea of pseudomembranous colitis due to a toxin produced by the anaerobe, *Clostridium difficile*
813   When this drug is taken for viral upper respiratory tract infection a macular rash is commonly seen
814   This drug shows a beneficial interaction with isoniazid, both being bactericidal to *Mycobacterium tuberculosis*

Options for 811–814:

    (A)   ampicillin
    (B)   benzylpenicillin [penicillin G]
    (C)   cloxacillin
    (D)   ethambutol
    (E)   metronidazole
    (F)   rifampicin [rifampin]

Select the natural substrate of which each chemotherapeutic agent is the closest structural analogue:

815   benzylpenicillin [penicillin G]
816   cephaloridine
817   cycloserine
818   dapsone (a sulphone)
819   methotrexate
820   pyrimethamine
821   sodium aminosalicylate
822   sulphadimidine
823   trimethoprim

Options for 815–823:

    (A)   D-alanine
    (B)   D-alanyl-D-alanine
    (C)   dihydrofolate
    (D)   *p*-aminobenzoate

Select the most appropriate treatment for infestation by each parasite:

824   roundworm (*Ascaris* sp.)
825   tapeworm (*Taenia* sp.)
826   threadworm (*Enterobius* sp.)

Options for 824–826:

    (A)   dichlorophen
    (B)   diethylcarbamazine
    (C)   niridazole
    (D)   piperazine

Select the drug most likely to cause toxic damage to:

827   inner ear (impaired balance and hearing)
828   bone marrow (aplastic anaemia)
829   kidney (crystalluria)

Options for 827–829:

    (A)   chloramphenicol
    (B)   chloroquine
    (C)   cycloserine
    (D)   isoniazid
    (E)   sodium aminosalicylate
    (F)   streptomycin
    (G)   sulphonamides
    (H)   tetracycline

Indicate the chemotherapy most appropriate to:

830   abolish the carrier state in typhoid fever
831   hasten recovery from mycoplasmal pneumonia
832   eradicate oropharyngeal candidiasis
833   treat an exacerbation of chronic bronchitis in a patient with mild chronic renal failure

Options for 830–833:

    (A)   parenteral gentamicin
    (B)   parenteral amphotericin
    (C)   oral ampicillin
    (D)   oral tetracycline
    (E)   none of A to D

Select the most appropriate tabulated description for each of the following penicillins:

834   amoxycillin
835   ampicillin
836   benzylpenicillin [penicillin G]
837   carbenicillin
838   cloxacillin
839   flucloxacillin

840 methicillin
841 phenoxymethylpenicillin [penicillin V]
842 procaine penicillin

Options for 834–842:

	Spectrum	Susceptibility to gastric acid	Susceptibility to Staphylococcal penicillinase
(A)	narrower	labile	labile
(B)	narrower	labile	stable
(C)	narrower	stable	labile
(D)	narrower	stable	stable
(E)	wider	labile	labile
(F)	wider	stable	labile

Select the best description of the mechanism of the toxic action on susceptible parasites of:

843 benzylpenicillin [penicillin G]
844 busulphan
845 cephaloridine
846 chloramphenicol
847 chlorhexidine
848 chloroquine
849 cycloserine
850 cytarabine
851 emetine
852 erythromycin
853 fluorouracil
854 fusidic acid
855 γ benzene hexachloride
856 hexachlorophane
857 idoxuridine
858 lincomycin
859 mercaptopurine
860 methotrexate
861 nitrogen mustards (e.g. mustine [mechlorethamine])
862 polyene antibiotics (e.g. nystatin)
863 polypeptide antibiotics (e.g. colistin)
864 pyrimethamine
865 quinine

866   sodium aminosalicylate
867   streptomycin
868   sulphonamides (e.g. sulphadimidine)
869   sulphones (e.g. dapsone)
870   tetracycline
871   trimethoprim

Options for 843–871:

  (A)   inhibition of cell wall synthesis
  (B)   inhibition of nucleic acid synthesis by reduced production of tetrahydrofolate
  (C)   inhibition of nucleic acid synthesis by competition with purines or pyrimidines
  (D)   inhibition of nucleic acid replication by combination with nucleic acid
  (E)   inhibition of protein synthesis by prevention of ribosomal binding of amino-acyl-*t*-RNA
  (F)   inhibition of protein synthesis by inhibition of ribosomal peptidyl transferase
  (G)   inhibition of protein synthesis by prevention of ribosomal translocation
  (H)   cytotoxic action by primary damage to the cell membrane

Type 8

872   Methotrexate overdosage is corrected by folic acid administration

  BECAUSE

  methotrexate competes with dihydrofolate for dihydrofolate hydrogenase

873   Some sulphonamides cause goitre and/or hypothyroidism

  BECAUSE

  some (the same) sulphonamides block iodide uptake by the thyroid gland

874   Some sulphonamides cause diuresis and acidification of the urine

  BECAUSE

  some (the same) sulphonamides are inhibitors of carbonic anhydrase

875 Some sulphonamides cause a lowering of blood sugar

BECAUSE

some (the same) sulphonamides cause release of endogenous insulin

876 Sulphamethoxazole and trimethoprim potentiate each other

BECAUSE

sulphamethoxazole and trimethoprim are both inhibitors of dihydrofolate synthetase

877 Tetracycline is deposited in newly forming teeth

BECAUSE

tetracycline chelates calcium ions

878 The antibacterial activity of a sulphonamide when applied to a bacterial culture *in vitro* is reduced if folic acid is added at the same time

BECAUSE

sulphonamides inhibit dihydrofolate synthetase

879 People who have the genetic abnormality of glucose-6-phosphate dehydrogenase deficiency are partially resistant to malaria

BECAUSE

the malarial parasite is partially dependent upon the functioning of the 'pentose shunt'

Type 9

880 The selective toxicity of each of the following chemotherapeutic agents depends on its selective distribution in the animal:

(A) chloroquine
(B) cyclophosphamide

    (C)   griseofulvin
    (D)   nalidixic acid
    (E)   nitrofurantoin

881 The following antibacterial drugs are useful against *Pseudomonas aeruginosa*:

    (A)   carbenicillin
    (B)   colistin
    (C)   erythromycin
    (D)   gentamicin

882 Sensitive bacteria are killed by the serum concentrations attained during clinical use of the following drugs:

    (A)   benzylpenicillin [penicillin G]
    (B)   cephaloridine
    (C)   streptomycin
    (D)   tetracycline

883 The following antibacterial drugs act by inhibiting cell wall synthesis:

    (A)   benzylpenicillin [penicillin G]
    (B)   cephaloridine
    (C)   cycloserine
    (D)   streptomycin

884 The following drugs act by inhibiting dihydrofolate hydrogenase:

    (A)   methotrexate
    (B)   pyrimethamine
    (C)   sulphadimidine
    (D)   trimethoprim

885 The following kinds of malignant disease often show a useful therapeutic response to cytotoxic drugs:

    (A)   carcinoma (e.g. of the colon)
    (B)   choriocarcinoma
    (C)   leukaemia
    (D)   lymphoma (e.g. Hodgkin's disease)

86 Sulphonamides:

    (A)   are structural analogues of *p*-aminobenzoic acid
    (B)   reduce the synthesis of dihydrofolate in susceptible bacteria
    (C)   do not reduce the synthesis of dihydrofolate in mammalian cells
    (D)   are oxidised in the liver to biologically inactive metabolites

87 The following drugs are useful in the treatment of intestinal amoebiasis:

    (A)   chloroquine
    (B)   emetine
    (C)   diloxanide
    (D)   metronidazole

88 The following drugs are useful in the treatment of hepatic amoebiasis:

    (A)   chloroquine
    (B)   emetine
    (C)   metronidazole
    (D)   tetracycline

89 The incidence of generalised vaccinia after smallpox vaccination is increased if the patient is receiving:

    (A)   methyldopa
    (B)   methotrexate
    (C)   prednisolone
    (D)   merceptopurine

90 A prodrug is relatively inactive itself but is converted to a more active drug within the body. The following chemotherapeutic agents are prodrugs:

    (A)   azathioprine
    (B)   cyclophosphamide
    (C)   malathion
    (D)   proguanil
    (E)   trimethoprim

6 Drug Disposition and Metabolism

Type 1

891 The long-acting sulphonamide, sulphadimethoxine, increases the risk of brain damage due to an excessive plasma concentration of free bilirubin in the newborn child. The sulphonamide:

(A) competes with bilirubin for plasma albumin binding sites
(B) inhibits hepatic glucuronyl transferase
(C) promotes the haemolysis of fetal red blood cells
(D) reduces the effectiveness of the blood brain barrier

892 Drug X competes with drug Y for the same binding sites on the plasma albumin molecule. When Y is administered alone 95% of the drug in plasma is protein-bound and the plasma concentration half-time is 4 hours. When X is administered simultaneously Y is 90% protein bound and the half-time of Y is approximately:

(A) 1 hour
(B) 2 hours
(C) 6 hours
(D) 8 hours

(Assume that the elimination of Y obeys first-order kinetics)

Figure 10 shows the relationship between the concentration *d* of drug free in the plasma water and the total concentration C_p in plasma.
Use this information for questions 893–896.

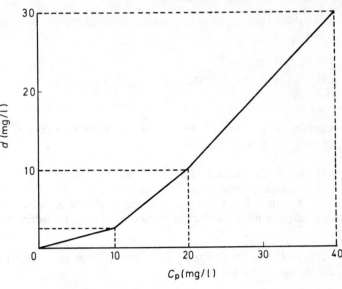

Figure 10

893 When C_p is below 10 mg/ℓ the proportion of drug which is protein-bound is approximately:

(A) 25%
(B) 50%
(C) 75%

894 The binding sites with the greatest affinity are virtually fully saturated when C_p equals approximately:

(A) 10 mg/ℓ
(B) 20 mg/ℓ
(C) 30 mg/ℓ
(D) 40 mg/ℓ

895 The binding sites with the least affinity are virtually fully saturated when C_p equals approximately:

(A) 10 mg/ℓ
(B) 20 mg/ℓ
(C) 30 mg/ℓ
(D) 40 mg/ℓ

896 The plasma concentration half-time of the drug is likely to be shortest when C_p is:

    (A)   below 10 mg/ℓ
    (B)   between 10 and 20 mg/ℓ
    (C)   above 20 mg/ℓ

897 Digoxin has a longer plasma concentration half-time than gentamicin because

    (A)   the renal clearance of digoxin is smaller
    (B)   digoxin is metabolised less rapidly
    (C)   digoxin is more extensively bound to plasma proteins
    (D)   digoxin has a much greater effective volume of distribution

898 Benzylpenicillin [penicillin G] has a shorter plasma concentration half-life than gentamicin because:

    (A)   the renal clearance of benzylpenicillin [penicillin G] is larger
    (B)   benzylpenicillin [penicillin G] is metabolised more rapidly
    (C)   benzylpenicillin [penicillin G] is less extensively bound to plasma proteins
    (D)   benzylpenicillin [penicillin G] has a smaller effective volume of distribution

899 The concurrent administration of phenobarbitone increases the dosage of warfarin required for effective anticoagulant therapy because:

    (A)   phenobarbitone displaces warfarin from albumin binding sites thus increasing the rate of elimination of warfarin
    (B)   phenobarbitone forms an inactive complex with warfarin
    (C)   phenobarbitone induces liver microsomal oxidase, thus increasing the rate of biotransformation of warfarin
    (D)   phenobarbitone diminishes the renal tubular reabsorption of warfarin

900 The equation which correctly describes the relationship between the plasma concentration half-time $T_{1/2}$ (min), the distribution volume V (mℓ) and the elimination clearance Cl (mℓ/min) of a drug is:

    (A) $T_{1/2} = 0.7\,V \times Cl$
    (B) $T_{1/2} = 0.7\,Cl/V$

(C) $T_{1/2} = 0.7 \ V/Cl$
(D) $T_{1/2} = 0.7(1/V) \times Cl$

901   The $T_{1/2}$ for digoxin in a patient of 70 kg ($V = 5000$ mℓ/kg) who has
digoxin clearance of 140 mℓ/min is:

$$T_{1/2} = \frac{0.7 \times 350000}{140}$$

(A)   1440 min (24 hours)
(B)   1750 min (about 29 hours)
(C)   2000 min (about 33 hours)
(D)   3500 min (about 58 hours)

902   The $T_{1/2}$ for digoxin in a patient of 70 kg ($V = 5000$ mℓ/kg) with severe
renal insufficiency who has digoxin clearance of 35 mℓ/min is:

(A)   3500 min (about 58 hours)
(B)   7000 min (about 116 hours)
(C)   10 000 min (about 166 hours)
(D)   14 000 min (about 232 hours)

903   The time required for induction of anaesthesia with a volatile agent is
dependent upon the partial pressure (P) of anaesthetic gas in the inspired air, the blood/gas partition coefficient (λ) and the body mass
(m). There is a positive linear relationship between this time and:

(A) $P\lambda m$
(B) $P\lambda/m$
(C) $P/\lambda m$
(D) $\lambda m/P$
(E) λ/mP
(F) $m/\lambda P$

904   The time required for recovery from prolonged anaesthesia due to a
volatile agent is dependent upon the duration of anaesthesia (T_a), the
body mass (m), the respiratory minute volume (R) and the blood/gas
partition coefficient (λ). There is a positive linear relation between this
time and:

(A) $T_a m\lambda/R$
(B) $T_a m/\lambda R$
(C) $T_a/m\lambda R$

    (D) $R/T_a m\lambda$
    (E) $RT_a/m\lambda$
    (F) $RT_a m/\lambda$

905 Ethanol is eliminated mainly by:

    (A)   excretion in the expired air
    (B)   excretion in the urine
    (C)   oxidation in the liver
    (D)   acetylation in the liver

906 Disulfiram interferes with the metabolism of ethanol by:

    (A)   inhibition of alcohol dehydrogenase
    (B)   inhibition of the mixed function oxidase of liver microsomes
    (C)   inhibition of aldehyde oxidase
    (D)   inhibition of alcohol acetylase

907 Nausea and wretchedness are produced by ethanol in the presence of disulfiram. The symptoms are due to the accumulation in the blood of:

    (A)   acetaldehyde
    (B)   acetate
    (C)   ethyl acetate
    (D)   formaldehyde

908 The part of the gut from which ethanol is absorbed earliest is the:

    (A)   stomach
    (B)   duodenum
    (C)   jejunum
    (D)   ileum

909 Ethanol (molecular weight 46) is absorbed rapidly from the gut because:

    (A)   it is a non-polar compound which is highly lipid-soluble
    (B)   it is a polar compound which is water-soluble and small enough to diffuse through water-filled pores in cell membranes
    (C)   it is absorbed by facilitated diffusion
    (D)   it is absorbed by 'uphill' transport

Figure 11 shows the relationship between the urinary pH and the ratio of the concentration of free drug in the urine (C_u) to the concentration of free drug in the plasma (C_p).
Use this information to answer questions 910–913.

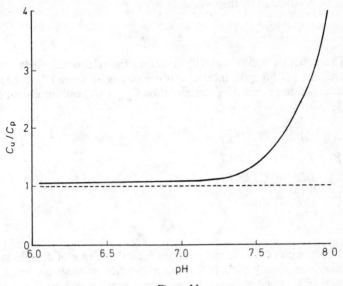

Figure 11

910 The drug is:

(A) a weak acid
(B) a weak base
(C) fully ionised over the pH range

911 The pK_a of the drug is:

(A) not deducible from the information given
(B) less than 8
(C) greater than 8

912 The diffusible form of the drug diffuses through the renal tubular epithelium:

(A) less rapidly than water
(B) more rapidly than water
(C) at the same rate as water

913   The plasma half-time of the drug is likely to be:

(A)   shortest when the urine is maximally alkaline
(B)   shortest when the urine is maximally acid
(C)   unaffected by the urine pH

914   The equation which correctly describes the relationship between the drug dose D (μg), the interval between successive doses T (h), the mean steady-state plasma drug concentration $\bar{C}_{pss}$ (μg/ℓ) and the clearance Cl (ℓ/h) is:

(A) $DT \ = \ \bar{C}_{pss} \times Cl$
(B) $T/D \ = \ \bar{C}_{pss} \times Cl$
(C) $D/T \ = \ \bar{C}_{pss} \times Cl$
(D) $D/T \ = \ \bar{C}_{pss} / Cl$

915   A child with cardiac failure develops clinical evidence of digitalis intoxication on a daily dose of 100 μg of digoxin as paediatric elixir. The mean steady-state plasma digoxin concentration is 4 μg/ℓ. Assuming complete absorption the elimination clearance of digoxin (ℓ/h) in this patient is approximately:

(A)   0.5
(B)   1
(C)   1.5
(D)   2

916   After equilibration of digoxin between blood plasma and tissues, the drug occupies an effective distribution volume of 5 ℓ/kg bodyweight. Calculate the maximum intravenous loading dose required for an acute cardiac emergency in a 35 kg child (Christopher Robin). The plasma concentration after equilibration should not exceed 2 μg/ℓ.

(A)   70 μg
(B)   150 μg
(C)   350 μg
(D)   500 μg

917 After further consultation it is decided to give the loading dose of digoxin to the child (Christopher Robin) by mouth using 125 μg tablets which are approximately 60% absorbed. The largest safe dose is:

(A) one tablet
(B) two tablets
(C) four tablets
(D) six tablets
(E) eight tablets

918 After the loading dose, the child (Christopher Robin) is given a daily maintenance dose of 250 μg of digoxin by mouth. Indicate the serum biochemical measurement which would be most useful as a warning of impaired elimination of digoxin:

(A) measurement of albumin concentration
(B) measurement of bilirubin concentration
(C) measurement of Ca^{2+} concentration
(D) measurement of creatinine concentration
(E) measurement of K^+ concentration

919 The daily dose of sodium warfarin taken by a patient has been carefully adjusted to obtain a stable thrombotest result of 10–15%. Indicate the interacting drug which is most likely to produce a dramatic increase in anticoagulant effect:

(A) aspirin 600 mg
(B) diazepam 10 mg
(C) ethanol 20 ml
(D) phenobarbitone 100 mg
(E) phenylbutazone 400 mg

920 The metabolism of drugs by mixed-function oxidase enzymes requires:

(A) O_2 and NAD^+
(B) O_2 and NADPH
(C) CO_2 and ADP
(D) CO_2 and NAD^+
(E) CO and NADPH

921   This drug is metabolised to a pharmacologically active derivative:

(A)   paracetamol [acetaminophen]
(B)   phenobarbitone
(C)   phenylbutazone
(D)   phenytoin [diphenylhydantoin]
(E)   sulphadimidine

922   Phenytoin [diphenylhydantoin] is eliminated from the body according to Michaelis-Menten kinetics. At low plasma concentrations, however, the elimination appears to be a first-order (exponential) process. The reduced form of the Michaelis-Menten equation applicable to the elimination of low plasma concentrations is:

(A) $dC_p/dt = -V_{max} + C_p/K_m + C_p$
(B) $dC_p/dt = -V_{max} C_p/K_m$
(C) $dC_p/dt = -K_m C_p/V_{max}$
(D) $dC_p/dt = -V_{max}$

where dC_p/dt = rate of change of plasma concentration C_p
V_{max} = theoretical maximum value of dC_p/dt
K_m = concentration at $V_{max}/2$

Type 2

Drugs differ in the extent to which they are absorbed from the gut. After the oral administration of:

923   amphetamine
924   antidiuretic hormone
925   atropine
926   atropine butylbromide
927   codeine
928   corticotrophin
929   cyloserine
930   ethanol
931   ephedrine
932   gentamicin
933   glyceryltrinitrate
934   hyoscine [scopolamine]
935   hyoscine [scopolamine] butylbromide
936   indomethacin

937   insulin
938   kanamycin
939   levodopa
940   lignocaine [lidocaine]
941   mannitol
942   methyldopa
943   neomycin
944   pempidine
945   benzylpenicillin [penicillin G]
946   pentolinium
947   phenylbutazone
948   propantheline bromide
949   quinidine
950   quinine
951   salicylic acid
952   streptomycin
953   tetraethylammonium
954   thyroxine
955   tubocurarine
956   warfarin

Options for 923–956

A large proportion of the dose reaches the systemic circulation by:

(A)   passive diffusion through the water-filled pores of the mucosal cell membrane

(B)   non-ionic diffusion through the lipid part of the mucosal cell membrane favoured by the relatively low pH of the stomach contents

(C)   non-ionic diffusion through the lipid part of the mucosal cell membrane favoured by the relatively high pH of the small bowel contents

(D)   carrier-mediated transport across the small bowel mucosa

Only a small proportion of the dose reaches the systemic circulation because the drug molecule:

(E)   although chemically stable *in vivo* is insoluble in lipid and penetrates the gut mucosa very slowly

(F)   is inactivated by the low pH of the stomach contents

(G)   is inactivated by gut peptidases

(H)   is inactivated in the liver before reaching the systemic circulation

Which of the sympathomimetic amine derivatives:

957 is least likely to be completely absorbed from the gut?

958 is most likely to be completely absorbed via the sublingual route?

959 is most likely to be absorbed from the gut and to show pH dependence of urinary excretion?

960 is most likely to have renal plasma clearance close to the glomerular filtration rate?

Options for 957–960:

Drugs enter the brain and cerebrospinal fluid at different rates. The drug:

961 amphetamine
962 barbitone
963 benzylpenicillin [penicillin G]
964 cycloserine
965 ethanol
966 levodopa
967 mannitol
968 methyldopa
969 pentolinium
970 streptomycin
971 thiopentone
972 tubocurarine

Options for 961–972:

(A) penetrates rapidly into the brain where the drug concentration rapidly approaches the concentration in the arterial blood plasma
(B) penetrates slowly into brain where the drug concentration slowly approaches the concentration in the arterial blood plasma
(C) may diffuse into cerebrospinal fluid but is actively removed by carrier-mediated transport
(D) enters cerebrospinal fluid and brain by carrier-mediated transport
(E) cannot diffuse into cerebrospinal fluid or brain

The pharmacological properties of a drug molecule are influenced by its physical state in solution in water. The degree of ionisation, the nature of the charge and the lipid solubility of the non-ionised form are important. Indicate the physical state in aqueous solution at pH 7.4 of:

973 acetylcholine
974 adrenaline [epinephrine]
975 amphetamine
976 atropine
977 atropine butyl bromide
978 physostigmine (eserine)
979 gallamine
980 gentamicin
981 heparin
982 hexobarbitone
983 hyoscine [scopolamine]
984 hyoscine [scopolamine] butyl bromide

985   isoprenaline [isoproterenol]
986   kanamycin
987   lignocaine [lidocaine]
988   mannitol
989   mecamylamine
990   neomycin
991   noradrenaline [norepinephrine]
992   pentolinium
993   phenytoin [diphenylhydantoin]
994   neostigmine
995   streptomycin
996   tetraethylammonium
997   thiopentone
998   tubocurarine
999   warfarin

Options for 973–999:

	Degree of ionisation	*Nature of charge*	*Non-ionised form: lipid-soluble*
(A)	complete	+/–	none
(B)	zero	none	no
(C)	partial	+	yes
(D)	partial	+	no
(E)	partial	–	yes
(F)	partial	–	no

The pharmacological effect of a drug may be terminated by a variety of processes. Indicate the process responsible for the termination of the following effects:

1000 anaesthesia due to an intravenous dose of thiobarbitone   *C*
1001 the cardiac action of digoxin   *B*
1002 hypertension due to an intravenous infusion of angiotensin amide   *A*
1003 pupil constriction due to ecothiopate [echothiophate]   *G*
1004 increased uterine activity due to oxytocin   *A*
1005 analgesia due to intramuscular morphine   *A*
1006 analgesia due to inhalation of nitrous oxide   *E*
1007 hypertension due to an intravenous infusion of noradrenaline [norepinephrine]   *D*
1008 antibacterial activity of serum due to an intravenous dose of streptomycin   *B*

1009 anaesthesia due to an intravenous dose of thiopentone C

1010 anticonvulsant effects of a single intravenous bolus dose of diazepam C

1011 antibacterial activity of serum due to an intramuscular dose of gentamicin B

1012 the anticonvulsant effect of oral phenytoin [diphenylhydantoin] A

1013 paralysis of skeletal muscle due to an intravenous dose of suxamethon-ium [succinylcholine] A

1014 paralysis of skeletal muscle due to an intravenous dose of tubocurarine B

Options for 1000–1014:

(A) biotransformation
(B) renal excretion of the unchanged drug
(C) redistribution into skeletal muscle or adipose tissue
(D) selective uptake into special storage sites
(E) excretion in the expired air
(F) repletion of the transmitter stores
(G) slow reactivation of inhibited enzymes or synthesis of new enzyme

The renal clearance of:

1015 acetanilide (pK$_a$ 0.3)
1016 amphetamine (pK$_a$ 9.9)
1017 benzylpenicillin [penicillin G] (pK$_a$ 2.8)
1018 phenobarbitone (pK$_a$ 7.4)
1019 quinine (pK$_a$ 8.6)
1020 salicylic acid (pK$_a$ 3.0)
1021 thiopentone (pK$_a$ 8.0)

Options for 1015–1021:

(A) is greatest in acid urine (pH 5)
(B) is greatest in alkaline urine (pH 8)
(C) is virtually independent of urine pH over the 5–8 range

A proportion of the dose of certain drugs persists in the body for a long time. Indicate the mechanism responsible for the persistence of each of the following drugs:

1022 arsenic
1023 chlorpromazine
1024 DDT

1025 lead
1026 mepacrine
1027 strontium
1028 tetracycline

Options for 1022–1028:

    (A) binding to nucleic acids in liver cell nuclei
    (B) formation of stable complexes with bone salt
    (C) replacement of calcium ion in bone salt
    (D) formation of stable linkages with sulphur-rich protein
    (E) high lipid solubility combined with a slow rate of biotransformation
    (F) enterohepatic recycling of the compound

Indicate the molecular form of the drug which is responsible for the following pharmacological effects:

1029 atropine inhibits the effects of cholinergic nerve stimulation
1030 physostigmine (eserine) inhibits cholinesterase
1031 parathion (an organophosphorus derivative) inhibits cholinesterase
1032 procaine inhibits propagation of an action potential along a nerve axon
1033 probenecid decreases the renal clearance of benzylpenicillin [penicillin G]

Options for 1029–1033:

    (A) the unionised form
    (B) the anionic form
    (C) the cationic form
    (D) a metabolic derivative

Indicate the place where most of the dose would be situated 8 hours after the administration of each of the following drugs to patients with normal cardio-respiratory function and normal kidney function:

1034 half a million units of benzylpenicillin [penicillin G] by intramuscular injection
1035 160 mg gentamicin by intramuscular injection
1036 500 μg of digoxin as tablets with rapid dissolution properties
1037 1 g of neomycin by mouth
1038 a dose of nitrous oxide sufficient to produce a brief period of analgesia

Options for 1034–1038:

(A) atmosphere
(B) urine in bladder or voided
(C) gut lumen
(D) extracellular fluid
(E) skeletal muscle
(F) body fat

During the metabolism of xenobiotics two types of biochemical reaction, known as Phase 1 (usually oxidation) and Phase 2 (usually conjugation) reactions, can occur. Which reactions do each of the following xenobiotics undergo:

1039 benzene
1040 gentamicin
1041 nitrous oxide
1042 phenol
1043 phenytoin [diphenylhydantoin]

Options for 1039–1043:

(A) Phase 1 reaction succeeded by a Phase 2 reaction
(B) Phase 1 reaction only
(C) Phase 2 reaction only
(D) neither Phase 1 nor Phase 2 reactions

Knowledge of serum drug concentration may help when deciding whether drug dosage is excessive or inadequate. Indicate the most appropriate time for the collection of blood serum when:

1044 digoxin intoxication is suspected in a patient with multiple ventricular ectopic beats
1045 a septicaemic patient is failing to respond to treatment with gentamicin
1046 a patient with severe chronic renal insufficiency is receiving a course of gentamicin treatment and further loss of kidney function could be life-threatening
1047 non-compliance is suspected in a patient with epilepsy for whom phenytoin [diphenylhydantoin] sodium has been prescribed

Options for 1044–1047:

   (A)   1 hour after dosage
   (B)   3 hours after dosage
   (C)   6 or more hours after dosage
   (D)   immediately before dosage
   (E)   time is not critical

Type 5

During long-term anticonvulsant therapy with (1048), the desired therapeutic serum concentration range of (1049) is often difficult to obtain due to the (1050) relationship between the steady-state serum concentration and the dose.

Options for 1048–1050:

1048 (A)   chlorpromazine
     (B)   diazepam
     (C)   phenytoin [diphenylhydantoin]
     (D)   thiopentone

1049 (A)   1–5 μg/ℓ
     (B)   5–10 μg/ℓ
     (C)   10–20 mg/ℓ
     (D)   20–40 mg/ℓ

1050 (A)   zero-order
     (B)   linear
     (C)   non-linear
     (D)   non-existent

When a drug is given to a patient at a fixed daily dosage rate a steady state eventually develops in which the mean plasma drug concentration (mg/l) does not change from day to day. This concentration, which is often a major determinant of the clinical response, is equal to the (1051) divided by the (1052); the concentration doubles when the daily dosage rate is doubled unless the drug is eliminated by (1053) mechanisms as typified by (1054). Generally, the time taken to attain a steady state is directly proportional to the (1055) and when the former is long, as in the case of (1056), it may be necessary to give a loading dose in order to obtain a rapid clinical response. The size of this dose is determined primarily by the size of the (1057) which can be very great, particularly in the case of very (1058) drug molecules. The size of the daily dose required to maintain a desired mean plasma drug concentration is however determined primarily by the (1059) which in the case of very water-soluble drugs is determined primarily by the (1060) of the individual patient.

Options for 1051–1060:

1051 (A) area (mg/ℓ × h) under the concentration against time curve
and   between doses
1052 (B) volume of distribution (ℓ)
(C) daily dosage rate (mg/24 h)
(D) interval between doses (h)
(E) plasma drug concentration half-time (h)

1053 (A) saturable
(B) unsaturable

1054 (A) digoxin
(B) gentamicin
(C) phenytoin [diphenylhydantoin]
(D) propranolol
(E) thiopentone

1055 (A) daily dosage rate (mg/24 h)
(B) plasma clearance (ℓ/h)
(C) interval between doses (h)
(D) mean plasma drug concentration (mg/ℓ)
(E) plasma drug concentration half-time (h)

1056 (A) benzylpenicillin [penicillin G]
(B) digoxin
(C) isoprenaline [isoproterenol]
(D) procainamide
(E) streptomycin

1057 (A) volume of distribution (ℓ)
(B) daily dosage rate (mg/24 h)
(C) plasma clearance (ℓ/h)
(D) plasma concentration half-time (h)

1058 (A) acidic
(B) fat-soluble
(C) large
(D) water-soluble

1059 (A)   volume of distribution (ℓ)
  (B)   plasma clearance (ℓ/h)
  (C)   interval between doses (h)
  (D)   plasma concentration half-life (h)

1060 (A)   body surface area (m²)
  (B)   glomerular filtration rate (ℓ/h)
  (C)   lean body mass (kg)
  (D)   liver blood flow rate (ℓ/h)
  (E)   liver weight (kg)

Consider a patient who absorbs the whole of a dose D (mg) of drug given every T hours; substantial accumulation occurs when the drug has a long elimination half-time $T_{1/2}$ (h). Eventually a steady state is reached in which the average amount of drug in the body $\overline{D}_{ss}$ (mg) exceeds the single dose D (mg) by a factor of (1061). In the case of phenobarbitone the half-time $T_{1/2}$ is approximately (1062) hours. Thus a patient who absorbs 30 mg every 8 hours eventually accumulates a total body phenobarbitone of about (1063) mg.

Options for 1061–1063:

1061 (A) $1.44\,(T_{1/2} - T)$
  (B) $1.44\,T_{1/2}/T$
  (C) $1.44\,T^2/T_{1/2}$
  (D) $1.44\,T_{1/2}/D \times T$

1062 (A)   12
  (B)   24
  (C)   72
  (D)   108

1063 (A)   130
  (B)   230
  (C)   390
  (D)   690

Type 9

1064 The rate of induction of anaesthesia by an inhalational agent is increased by:

  (A)   a high alveolar ventilation rate
  (B)   a high anaesthetic potency

(C)   a high partial pressure of anaesthetic in inspired air
(D)   a high tissue/gas solubility coefficient ×
(E)   a low body mass

1065 The total quantity of an inhalational anaesthetic present in the body of a patient at the point of just recovering consciousness after a period of anaesthesia is high when:

(A)   the body mass is high
(B)   the period of exposure to anaesthetic was long
(C)   the potency of the anaesthetic is high
(D)   the tissue/gas solubility coefficient is high

7 Applied Pharmacology

Type 1

1066 The absorption of levodopa from the intestine is impaired by:

(A) dopa decarboxylase inhibitors
(B) dopamine
(C) monoamine oxidase inhibitors
(D) tyrosine

1067 Of the following agents, which is the most effective for the relief of a migrainous attack:

(A) aspirin
(B) caffeine
(C) ergometrine
(D) ergotamine tartrate
(E) indomethacin
(F) 100% oxygen

1068 Retroperitoneal fibrosis is a hazard following therapy with:

(A) propranolol
(B) methysergide
(C) tyramine
(D) progesterone
(E) clonidine

1069 The annual incidence of admission to hospital due to self-poisoning in the UK per 1000 of the adult population is:

(A) 0.1
(B) 1
(C) 10
(D) 100

1070 The annual death rate due to self-poisoning in the UK as a proportion of the death rate due to road traffic accidents is approximately:

(A) 0.5%
(B) 1%
(C) 2%
(D) 4%

1071 When treating a patient with severe oral barbiturate poisoning the highest priority must be given to:

(A) emptying the stomach and binding unabsorbed drug residues
(B) assisting elimination of the unchanged barbiturate by alkalinisation of the urine
(C) maintaining a clear airway and adequate lung ventilation
(D) increasing venous return and cardiac output by the intravenous infusion of fluid
(E) prophylactic antibiotic therapy
(F) increasing the arterial blood pressure by intravenous administration of pressor amines

1072 An epileptic patient receiving 300 mg phenytoin [diphenylhydantoin] daily discovers one evening that he has forgotten to take his morning and mid-day doses (100 mg each). He should:

(A) omit these doses completely and proceed with his usual evening dose
(B) take the total daily dose of 300 mg that evening
(C) take his usual evening dose and spread the missed doses over the next 48 hours

1073 When treating a patient with severe poisoning due to an organophos
phorus insecticide the highest priority must be given to:

(A) measurement of serum cholinesterase activity
(B) reactivation of cholinesterase by the intravenous administration
of pralidoxime
(C) inhibition of salivation, bronchial secretion and bradycardia by
the injection of atropine
(D) inhibition of skeletal muscle fasciculation by the injection of
tubocurarine

1074 The maximum incidence of (non-therapeutic) drug ingestion in chil
dren is found in the following group:

(A) boys aged 5–10 years
(B) boys aged 1–3 years
(C) girls aged 5–10 years
(D) girls aged 1–3 years

1075 As used in rheumatoid arthritis which of the following medicaments
is associated with the least incidence of *serious* toxic effects:

(A) aspirin
(B) chloroquine
(C) indomethacin
(D) penicillamine
(E) phenylbutazone
(F) prednisolone
(G) sodium aurothiomalate [gold sodium thiomalate]

1076 Congestive cardiac failure is characterised by:

(A) low cardiac output
(B) raised central venous pressure
(C) low resting (end-diastolic) ventricular pressure

1077 The hypotensive drug which is most likely to cause troublesome pos
tural (orthostatic) hypotension is:

(A) chlorthalidone

(B)   guanethidine
(C)   hydrallazine
(D)   propranolol

1078 The hypotensive drug with the least component of action on the central nervous system is:

(A)   clonidine
(B)   guanethidine
(C)   methyldopa
(D)   propranolol

1079 Malarial headache is best treated by:

(A)   chloroquine
(B)   diazepam
(C)   indomethacin
(D)   phenylbutazone
(E)   primaquine

1080 The toxicity of digoxin may be increased by administration of:

(A)   amiloride
(B)   frusemide [furosemide]
(C)   oral slow-release potassium chloride
(D)   spironolactone

1081 Pernicious anaemia should be treated initially with:

(A)   blood transfusion
(B)   ferrous sulphate
(C)   folic acid
(D)   hydroxycobalamin

1082 Among the treatments which aid the spontaneous healing of gastric ulcers is the use of:

(A)   calcium carbonate
(B)   carbenoxolone

(C)   propantheline
(D)   sodium bicarbonate

1083 Treatment of severe diarrhoea in neonates lasting for several days cc
include the use of:

(A)   diphenoxylate
(B)   intravenous dextrose and sodium chloride
(C)   methylcellulose
(D)   neomycin

1084 The least harmful anorectic is:

(A)   amphetamine
(B)   diethylpropion
(C)   fenfluramine
(D)   mazindol
(E)   phentermine

Type 2

Select the best treatment for each of the following conditions:

1085 atrial fibrillation with high ventricular rate
1086 heart failure due to beriberi
1087 cor pulmonale
1088 hypertensive encephalopathy
1089 prevention of migraine
1090 phaeochromocytoma
1091 pulmonary venous congestion

Options for 1085–1091:

(A)   clonidine
(B)   diazoxide
(C)   digoxin
(D)   frusemide [furosemide] (intravenously)
(E)   oxygen (by mask)
(F)   phenoxybenzamine and propranolol
(G)   thiamine

Select the dominant mechanism of action of each antiasthmatic drug:

1092 adrenaline [epinephrine]
1093 aminophylline
1094 choline theophyllinate
1095 sodium cromoglycate [cromolyn sodium]
1096 ephedrine
1097 hydrocortisone
1098 isoprenaline [isoproterenol]
1099 orciprenaline [metaproterenol]
1100 salbutamol

Options for 1092–1100:

(A)   prevention of the formation or release of active mediators of bronchoconstriction induced by challenge with allergen
(B)   specific competitive antihistamine effect
(C)   functional antagonism of the mediators by an indirect sympathomimetic mechanism
(D)   functional antagonism of the mediators by an agonist action at adrenoceptors
(E)   functional antagonism of the mediators by a direct relaxant effect on bronchiolar smooth muscle cells
(F)   non-specific suppression of inflammatory responses

Select one drug which:

1101 is effective for the immediate suppression of a series of grand mal convulsions but only when given intravenously
1102 has been shown experimentally to lower the serum concentration of phenytoin [diphenylhydantoin] when given to patients receiving a fixed dose of phenytoin
1103 is partially metabolised to phenobarbitone in man
1104 is eliminated more rapidly when the urine pH is raised to 8.
1105 is effective against petit mal but not grand mal epilepsy
1106 on prolonged administration causes hyperplasia of the gums which become prominent and bleed easily

Options for 1101–1106:

(A)   diazepam
(B)   phenobarbitone

    (C)   phenytoin [diphenylhydantoin]
    (D)   primidone
    (E)   troxidone

Select an anticonvulsant which:

1107 is effective in status epilepticus but can cause local tissue necrosis when the drug has been partially oxidised during storage
1108 can cause ataxia, dysarthria (difficulty in speech) and nystagmus (flickering eye movements), without clouding of consciousness, at serum concentrations of 25–35 μg/mℓ
1109 is effective in petit mal epilepsy
1110 can cause a folate-responsive megaloblastic anaemia

Options for 1107–1110:

    (A)   ethosuximide
    (B)   paraldehyde
    (C)   phenobarbitone
    (D)   phenytoin [diphenylhydantoin]
    (E)   primidone

In bronchial asthma which drug:

1111 is usually contraindicated because of its depressant action on the respiratory centre?
1112 competitively antagonises endogenous catecholamines at the β-receptors on cardiac muscle but has less effect on the bronchial β-receptors?
1113 may precipitate an attack of asthma in an atopic subject?
1114 is effective in producing bronchial relaxation but whose frequent use may precipitate cardiac arrhythmias?
1115 revents the release of the pharmacological mediators of the immune esponse?

Options for 1111–1115:

    (A)   ephedrine
    (B)   isoprenaline [isoproterenol]
    (C)   mepyramine
    (D)   morphine
    (E)   practolol
    (F)   prednisolone

(G)   propranolol
(H)   sodium cromoglycate [cromolyn sodium]

Indicate the binding or complexing agent most suitable for the treatment of poisoning by oral:

1116 digoxin
1117 glutethimide
1118 hyoscine [scopolamine]
1119 imipramine
1120 iron salts
1121 lead salts
1122 mercury salts
1123 paraquat
1124 phenobarbitone
1125 salicylic acid

Options for 1116–1125:

(A)   oral activated charcoal
(B)   intravenous calcium citrate
(C)   intravenous calcium edetate
(D)   intramuscular dimercaprol
(E)   intramuscular desferrioxamine
(F)   oral Fuller's earth

Indicate the drug which, in cases of acute poisoning, is most likely to produce each of the following sets of clinical features:

1126 overventilation, sweating and rapid pulse rate
1127 ulceration of the lips and tongue, damage to kidney and liver and death from progressive pulmonary fibrosis
1128 early features suggestive of acute alcohol intoxication followed by acute renal failure
1129 fast pulse rate, fixed dilated pupils, confusion and hallucinations
1130 impaired consciousness, very low frequency of breathing and CO_2 retention in the blood

Options for 1126–1130:

(A)   aspirin
(B)   atropine

(C)   glycol antifreeze
(D)   morphine
(E)   paraquat
(F)   phenobarbitone

Select the anticonvulsant which:

1131 acts by inhibiting carbonic anhydrase
1132 when administered for 1 week before the menstrual period can reduce sodium and fluid retention and sometimes prevent associated grand mal convulsions
1133 also stabilises membrane potentials of cardiac cells and is sometimes used to suppress ventricular ectopic rhythms
1134 selectively benefits patients with the transient cerebral dysrhythmia which is associated with a spike and wave EEG complex
1135 is partially oxidised to an irritant acid when stored inappropriately
1136 is partially metabolised to phenobarbitone

Options for 1131–1136:

(A)   acetazolamide
(B)   ethosuximide
(C)   paraldehyde
(D)   phenobarbitone
(E)   phenytoin [diphenylhydantoin]
(F)   prednisolone
(G)   primidone

Indicate the drug which, in cases of acute poisoning, is most likely to produce each of the following sets of clinical features:

1137 circulatory arrest due to cardiac asystole occurring within 1 or 2 days of the overdose
1138 liver necrosis occurring within 2 or 3 days of the overdose
1139 acute inflammation of the fine respiratory passages
1140 nausea, vomiting and a very slow pulse rate
1141 deep unconsciousness, depressed breathing, depressed reflexes, diminished response to pain, depressed circulation and dilated pupils

Options for 1137–1141:

(A)   digoxin

(B)   hydrocarbon fuels
(C)   morphine
(D)   paracetamol [acetaminophen]
(E)   pentobarbitone
(F)   slow-release potassium chloride

A patient with grand mal epilepsy has been recommended to take phenytoin [diphenylhydantoin] sodium at a dose of 300 mg daily during the last 6 months. Convulsions are still occurring at the rate of about one per week and he is admitted for reassessment. Indicate the appropriate response when his serum concentration of phenytoin [diphenylhydantoin] on 2 consecutive days is found to be close to:

1142 2 μg/ml
1143 10 μg/ml
1144 15 μg/ml
1145 35 μg/ml

Options for 1142–1145:

(A)   try to ascertain why the patient is taking less than the recommended dose
(B)   increase the dose by 50 mg daily
(C)   increase the dose by 100 mg daily
(D)   make no change in dose but add another anticonvulsant drug
(E)   reduce the dose of phenytoin [diphenylhydantoin] and add another anticonvulsant drug

Select the appropriate drug:

1146 has a vasodilator action selective for the arterial tree and may therefore precipitate angina pectoris
1147 is only of prophylactic value in angina pectoris
1148 has a vasodilator action; is useful for the prevention of angina precipitated by exertion
1149 in controlled trials is no better than placebo in preventing angina pectoris

Options for 1146–1149:

(A)   glyceryl trinitrate
(B)   hydrallazine

    (C)   pentaerythritol tetranitrate
    (D)   propranolol

Select one drug which:

1150 inhibits gastric acid secretion and produces a dry mouth
1151 inhibits gastric acid secretion and does not produce a dry mouth
1152 does not inhibit gastric acid secretion and can produce oedema
1153 does not inhibit gastric acid secretion and produces constipation

Options for 1150–1153:

    (A)   aluminium hydroxide
    (B)   carbenoxolone sodium
    (C)   cimetidine
    (D)   dicyclomine
    (E)   magnesium hydroxide

Type 3

In questions 1154–1155 answer:

    (A)   if options I and II are appropriate
    (B)   if options I and III are appropriate
    (C)   if options I and IV are appropriate
    (D)   if options II and III are appropriate
    (E)   if options II and IV are appropriate
    (F)   if options III and IV are appropriate

1154 Caffeine:
    (I)   dilates cerebral blood vessels
    (II)   constricts cerebral blood vessels
    (III)   enhances absorption of ergot alkaloids from the gastrointestinal tract
    (IV)   decreases absorption of ergot alkaloids from the gastrointestinal tract

1155 In the initial stages of a migrainous attack there is:

    (I)   extracranial vasoconstriction

(II)   intracranial vasoconstriction
(III) extracranial vasodilation
(IV) intracranial vasodilation

Type 4

1156 Administration may cause extrapyramidal side-effects which resemble parkinsonism
1157 Necessitates an amine-free diet by the patient
1158 Is used primarily as a hypnotic
1159 Combines tranquillising and antidepressant properties

Options for 1156–1159:

(A) the tricyclic compound doxapine
(B) the monoamine oxidase inhibitor phenelzine
(C) the benzodiazepine nitrazepam
(D) the fluorinated phenothiazine trifluoperazine

Type 5

The principal action of digoxin in alleviating heart failure with sinus rhythm is (1160). If the failure is associated with atrial fibrillation and a rapid ventricular rate another action of digoxin (1161) is therapeutically useful.

The diuretic (1162) can precipitate digoxin toxicity. Digoxin toxicity may also result from the use of the potent diuretic ethacrynic acid. Continuous use of such diuretics increases (1163) and hence aggravates potassium depletion

Aminophylline and digoxin share the therapeutic action of (1164) and also share the toxic effect of (1165)

Options for 1160–1165:

1160 (A)   increased vagal activity and depression of conduction through the
and   atrioventricular node
1161 (B)   increased automaticity
     (C)   direct stimulation of the myocardium
     (D)   increased myocardial oxygen consumption

1162 (A)   amiloride
     (B)   frusemide [furosemide]
     (C)   spironolactone
     (D)   triamterene

1163 (A) acidosis
     (B) diabetes mellitus
     (C) gout
     (D) hyperaldosteronism
     (E) hypertension

1164 (A) bronchodilation
     (B) central nervous system stimulation
     (C) depression of cardiac contraction
     (D) increased renal blood flow

1165 (A) convulsions
     (B) heart block
     (C) hypotension
     (D) ventricular tachycardia

(1166) is a predominant symptom in most forms of neurotic illness and (1167), which acts selectively upon central (1168) systems, may relieve it. Neurosis is essentially of (1169) origin. Hospitalisation is (1170) needed and prognosis for recovery with treatment is good.

Options for 1166–1170:

1166 (A) anxiety
     (B) tremor
     (C) excitement
     (D) paralysis

1167 (A) amitriptyline
     (B) *l*-amphetamine
     (C) *d*-amphetamine
     (D) diazepam

1168 (A) cerebellar
     (B) cortical
     (C) limbic
     (D) medullary

 169 (A) biochemical
     (B) allergic
     (C) environmental
     (D) hereditary

1170 (A) always
     (B) frequently
     (C) seldom
     (D) never

Type 6

1171 (X) net water absorption in the colon in a person with diarrhoea
     (Y) net water absorption in the colon in a person without diarrhoea

1172 (X) rate of onset of laxative action of magnesium sulphate
     (Y) rate of onset of laxative action of methylcellulose

Type 8

1173 Diazepam is effective in treating mild depressive
     illness

   BECAUSE

   benzodiazepines stimulate the reticular formation

1174 Amitriptyline effectively controls nocturnal
     enuresis in children

   BECAUSE

   tricyclic antidepressants cause release of antidiuretic
   hormone from the anterior pituitary

1175 Butyrophenones cause side-effects which resemble
     Parkinson's disease

   BECAUSE

   butyrophenones stimulate cerebellar
   α-adrenoceptors

1176 Electroconvulsive therapy (ECT) is effective in
     endogenous depression

   BECAUSE

   ECT increases the rate of noradrenaline
   [norepinephrine] synthesis in the brain

1177 Meprobamate causes nocturnal restlessness

BECAUSE

meprobamate stimulates peripheral nicotinic
receptors

Type 9

1178 The neuromuscular blocking action of tubocurarine is potentiated by:

(A) penicillin
(B) ether
(C) neomycin
(D) polymixin
(E) streptomycin

1179 Tranylcypromine:

(A) increases the duration of action of pethidine [meperidine]
(B) enhances the activity of tyramine
(C) enhances the activity of phenylpropylamine
(D) enhances the activity of neostigmine

1180 The hypotensive effect of guanethidine can be antagonised by:

(A) amitriptyline
(B) bethanidine
(C) ephedrine
(D) imipramine

1181 Warfarin may be displaced from binding sites on plasma proteins by:

(A) phenobarbitone
(B) phenylbutazone
(C) sulphamethoxypyridazine
(D) sulphinpyrazone
(E) tolbutamide

182 Warfarin-metabolising enzymes in the liver are induced by:

   (A)   amylobarbitone
   (B)   dichloralphenazone
   (C)   nitrazepam
   (D)   phenobarbitone
   (E)   phenytoin [diphenylhydantoin]

183 A drug which is of value in the prophylaxis of migraine is:

   (A)   clonidine
   (B)   cyproheptadine
   (C)   methysergide
   (D)   phentolamine
   (E)   salicylate

184 Clonidine:

   (A)   is an imidazoline derivative
   (B)   diminishes responses of peripheral blood vessels to dilator stimuli
   (C)   diminishes responses of peripheral vessels to constrictor stimuli
   (D)   can cause hypotension
   (E)   is a potent antagonist of 5-hydroxytryptamine

185 In the treatment of osteoarthritis each of the following drugs could be prescribed as the drug of first choice:

   (A)   flufenamic acid
   (B)   ibuprofen
   (C)   indomethacin
   (D)   mefenamic acid
   (E)   phenylbutazone

186 In an attack of bronchial asthma of moderate severity:

   (A)   the timed forced expiratory volume (FEV_1) is reduced
   (B)   the partial pressure of CO_2 in arterial blood is high
   (C)   the partial pressure of O_2 in arterial blood is low
   (D)   the residual lung volume is increased

1187 A suitable treatment for a patient suffering mild asthmatic attacks is:

    (A)   aminophylline orally
    (B)   sodium cromoglycate [cromolyn sodium] by inhalation
    (C)   prednisolone orally
    (D)   terbutaline by inhalation

1188 A suitable treatment for a patient suffering moderate asthmatic attac
     is:

    (A)   beclomethasone by inhalation
    (B)   mepyramine orally
    (C)   prednisolone orally
    (D)   salbutamol by inhalation

1189 A suitable treatment for status asthmaticus is:

    (A)   aminophylline by intravenous injection
    (B)   diazepam orally
    (C)   hydrocortisone by intravenous injection
    (D)   salbutamol by inhalation

1190 Morphine may be given in acute left ventricular failure to:

    (A)   relieve pain
    (B)   relieve bronchospasm
    (C)   allay anxiety
    (D)   relieve dyspnoea

1191 Drugs useful in the immediate treatment of a hypertensive emergency
     complicated by pulmonary oedema include:

    (A)   diazoxide
    (B)   frusemide [furosemide]
    (C)   methyldopa
    (D)   sodium nitroprusside

1192 The value of propranolol in the treatment of hypertension is un-
doubted. Its site and mechanism of action are unclear. Tenable hypo-
theses include:

(A) antagonism of the neurotransmitter noradrenaline [norepine-
phrine] and the hormone adrenaline [epinephrine] at β-adrenoceptors in the heart
(B) antagonism of the neurotransmitter noradrenaline [norepine-
phrine] and the hormone adrenaline [epinephrine] at β-adrenoceptors in blood vessels
(C) modulation of the central (brain stem) integration of baro-
receptor reflexes
(D) inhibition of renin release from the kidney

1193 Administration of potassium citrate to change the urinary pH favours
excretion of:

(A) aspirin
(B) chloroquine
(C) nalidixic acid
(D) nitrofurantoin
(E) phenobarbitone

1194 Rational therapy for tension headache may include:

(A) aspirin
(B) gold salts
(C) nitrazepam
(D) paracetamol [acetaminophen]
(E) psychotherapy

1195 Damage to the embryo can be caused by:

(A) cyclophosphamide
(B) passive immunisation against rubella
(C) thalidomide
(D) irradiation of the pelvis with x-rays

1196 Motion sickness is controlled by:

- (A) chlorpromazine
- (B) cyclizine
- (C) hyoscine [scopolamine]
- (D) metoclopramide

1197 The following drugs are keratolytic:

- (A) clioquinol
- (B) resorcinol
- (C) salicylic acid
- (D) sulphur

1198 The following antibiotics commonly precipitate sensitisation when applied to the skin:

- (A) ampicillin
- (B) chlortetracycline
- (C) gentamicin
- (D) streptomycin

1199 Each of these drugs is useful in reducing the frequency and severity of relapses in patients with ulcerative colitis:

- (A) carbenoxolone
- (B) prednisolone
- (C) sulphasalazine

1200 Chlorpromazine produces:

- (A) sedation
- (B) suppression of abnormal behaviour in schizophrenia
- (C) elevation of mood in endogenous depression
- (D) suppression of vomiting due to morphine
- (E) suppression of symptoms of the alcohol withdrawal syndrome

Answers and Facilities of the Questions

Autonomic pharmacology

1	B	35	2	A	97	3	B	89	4	C	85
5	C	90	6	G	51	7	C	46	8	A	50
9	D	35	10	D	15	11	F	71	12	G	53
13	D	73	14	D	39	15	C	85	16	D	34
17	D	25	18	D	43	19	B	86	20	C	72
21	C	79	22	E	36	23	C	80	24	F	38
25	B	73	26	C	51	27	D	93	28	A	22
29	B	71	30	B	63	31	B	20	32	C	64
33	C	42	34	D	19	35	B	53	36	B	43
37	A	62	38	B	43	39	A	54	40	B	70
41	A	82	42	A	88	43	B	91	44	C	74
45	C	44	46	C	88	47	A	81	48	C	71
49	D	91	50	A	26	51	B	21	52	C	53
53	C	37	54	C	75	55	D	59	56	B	95
57	G	91	58	I	78	59	D	28	60	B	63
61	E	77	62	C	81	63	F	72	64	B	57
65	C	60	66	A	43	67	C	43	68	E	79
69	D	88	70	A	54	71	A	97	72	D	97
73	F	91	74	I	92	75	A	78	76	A	42
77	A	69	78	B	33	79	E	70	80	A	50
81	C	64	82	C	34	83	C	45	84	D	72
85	A	82	86	A	62	87	B	52	88	C	38
89	C	42	90	D	47	91	E	52	92	E	62
93	H	50	94	B	83	95	A	10	96	B	48
97	B	60	98	B	9	99	C	76	100	C	82
101	D	72	102	C	39	103	D	24	104	D	84
105	A	50	106	A	44	107	C	76	108	F	71

109	B	30	110	D	54	111	D	43	112	B	35
113	A	53	114	B	30	115	D	54	116	B	18
117	D	36	118	B	25	119	D	42	120	C	71
121	A	58	122	D	80	123	B	18	124	D	30
125	E	77	126	F	71	127	G	48	128	B	57
129	A	67	130	E	15	131	H	26	132	C	33
133	F	61	134	A	29	135	E	35	136	A	73
137	C	47	138	A	67	139	B	68	140	A	75
141	B	73	142	A	41	143	E	95	144	C	48
145	D	56	146	C	37	147	D	49	148	B	38
149	A	37	150	C	53	151	D	22	152	E	64
153	A	76	154	A	47	155	E	37	156	B	26
157	G	17	158	C	19	159	B	39	160	D	17
161	A	75	162	G	75	163	C	–	164	F	41
165	D	60	166	B	64	167	A	81	168	B	83
169	C	44	170	A	56	171	A	84	172	C	66
173	A	62	174	C	57	175	C	51	176	A	64
177	A	78	178	C	54	179	A	54	180	A	62
181	A	42	182	C	73	183	A	74	184	B	74
185	C	85	186	B	54	187	D	70	188	D	18
189	C	56	190	B	85	191	D	68	192	D	81
193	D	51	194	D	67	195	B	48	196	A	69
197	C	75	198	C	77	199	B	63	200	C	86
201	C	81									

Endocrine pharmacology

202	C	68	203	C	49	204	D	–	205	D	–
206	B	–	207	B	91	208	B	88	209	B	93
210	C	58	211	C	16	212	B	72	213	D	37
214	D	43	215	B	86	216	B	41	217	G	92
218	A	95	219	C	88	220	D	89	221	E	95
222	D	95	223	B	91	224	C	91	225	F	91
226	E	95	227	E	77	228	F	83	229	G	28
230	B	58	231	A	54	232	B	47	233	B	60
234	E	54	235	C	52	236	C	72	237	D	70
238	A	77	239	B	72	240	E	87	241	D	–
242	F	–	243	B	–	244	A	–	245	D	63
246	C	49	247	A	60	248	D	39	249	B	91
250	D	34	251	A	32	252	A	61	253	C	31
254	D	63	255	D	32	256	B	86	257	A	96
258	D	91	259	C	67	260	C	–	261	A	–
262	B	–	263	D	–	264	B	–	265	B	76

266	C	46	267	D	70	268	D	36	269	C	43
270	B	96	271	D	89	272	A	81	273	B	44
274	B	85	275	A	82	276	B	—	277	D	—
278	C	—	279	C	—	280	D	—	281	A	38
282	B	81	283	A	95	284	A	74	285	A	89
286	A	73	287	C	88	288	B	30	289	B	52
290	D	74	291	A	40	292	A	70	293	C	93
294	D	73	295	C	89	296	A	83	297	D	79
298	D	69	299	D	99	300	A	93	301	A	100
302	A	96	303	C	65	304	B	81	305	C	96
306	A	98	307	B	98	308	A	98	309	B	89
310	A	33	311	A	37	312	A	48	313	C	83
314	A	80	315	A	49	316	A	44	317	A	38
318	C	75	319	A	91	320	C	78	321	B	90
322	A	63	323	A	66	324	A	45	325	C	3
326	C	69	327	C	76	328	B	62	329	A	—
330	A	94	331	A	70	332	A	49	333	B	—
334	A	—	335	B	67	336	B	—	337	C	50
338	C	77	339	A	92	340	A	80	341	B	—
342	A	—	343	A	91	344	B	59	345	A	35
346	D	70	347	B	19	348	C	—	349	D	48
350	A	71	351	C	66	352	E	45	353	C	—
354	C	78	355	A	56	356	A	65	357	D	62
358	B	30	359	A	—	360	D	68	361	C	34
362	C	80	363	B	59	364	D	44	365	A	68
366	C	63	367	D	58	368	D	61	369	A	69
370	C	65	371	E	81	372	A	84	373	A	52
374	E	64	375	C	28	376	C	47	377	D	66
378	B	48	379	B	91	380	B	—	381	D	—
382	C	61	383	B	74	384	C	—	385	C	21
386	D	34	387	A	49	388	A	—	389	C	46
390	C	—	391	D	—	392	E	30	393	B	50
394	B	46	395	B	50	396	C	17	397	C	97
398	D	75	399	C	59	400	D	100	401	C	95
402	C	70	403	D	73	404	B	11			

Reproductive pharmacology

405	C	66	406	A	53	407	D	62	408	E	58
409	A	48	410	D	89	411	D	69	412	B	84
413	A	29	414	D	—	415	E	—	416	D	15
417	B	53	418	C	—	419	A	69	420	D	57
421	C	—	422	E	56	423	D	82	424	C	33

No.			No.			No.			No.		
425	C	—	426	D	80	427	A	43	428	B	10
429	B	—	430	F	78	431	E	71	432	A	78
433	G	88	434	C	96	435	E	76	436	D	92
437	B	69	438	A	10	439	C	32	440	C	32
441	B	—	442	B	—	443	C	—	444	B	—
445	E	67	446	B	70	447	C	80	448	F	24
449	D	59	450	C	66	451	B	31	452	E	56
453	F	49	454	E	51	455	A	94	456	A	48
457	B	75	458	C	57	459	C	96	460	B	62
461	C	15	462	B	58	463	A	—	464	C	14
465	C	78	466	D	86	467	A	76	468	B	83
469	D	88	470	E	93	471	A	81	472	F	85
473	C	74	474	C	84	475	C	42	476	A	58
477	C	74	478	B	63	479	A	—	480	C	—
481	D	—	482	B	—	483	D	89	484	E	85
485	C	99	486	B	84	487	A	86	488	B	—
489	D	—	490	E	—	491	A	—	492	C	89
493	A	88	494	B	89	495	B	61	496	A	63
497	D	66	498	C	79	499	D	82	500	B	41
501	B	71	502	C	72	503	C	54	504	C	35
505	A	84	506	A	91	507	C	96	508	D	61
509	B	76	510	B	90	511	B	47	512	C	86
513	A	86	514	D	89	515	C	96	516	A	93
517	A	86	518	B	69	519	D	44	520	A	73
521	C	63	522	A	78	523	B	39	524	B	93
525	C	25	526	C	32	527	D	—	528	A	—
529	D	—	530	A	—	531	D	—	532	C	17
533	C	63	534	C	77	535	A	33	536	C	81
537	C	—	538	C	58	539	C	91	540	C	—
541	C	—	542	A	—	543	C	—	544	A	47
545	A	—	546	C	—	547	A	—	548	A	56
549	C	—	550	C	61	551	A	—	552	C	66
553	A	—	554	A	47	555	A	64	556	D	—
557	B	63	558	E	60	559	A	—	560	E	—
561	B	—	562	E	—	563	A	79	564	E	—
565	C	—	566	C	—	567	A	24	568	D	15
569	B	28	570	D	42	571	C	38	572	A	—
573	D	—	574	A	—	575	D	—	576	D	46
577	D	25	578	C	39	579	C	—	580	A	71
581	C	80	582	B	53	583	C	60	584	C	—
585	F	—	586	B	17	587	C	31	588	A	46
589	A	—	590	C	65	591	C	41	592	E	—
593	B	—	594	E	—	595	C	73	596	E	23

Central nervous system pharmacology

597	C	—	598	B	50	599	A	80	600	C	47
601	E	92	602	B	30	603	A	56	604	C	65
605	A	34	606	C	65	607	B	39	608	D	55
609	A	28	610	A	26	611	A	48	612	D	89
613	A	64	614	C	72	615	E	66	616	B	60
617	B	63	618	C	56	619	C	63	620	A	—
621	E	—	622	C	—	623	E	—	624	D	—
625	B	—	626	C	—	627	D	78	628	F	49
629	B	35	630	A	—	631	D	62	632	B	63
633	G	40	634	A	55	635	G	26	636	C	65
637	F	16	638	E	39	639	A	57	640	G	59
641	D	7	642	A	63	643	D	56	644	E	51
645	F	91	646	C	—	647	A	—	648	D	—
649	B	—	650	C	67	651	B	46	652	A	49
653	D	45	654	C	86	655	B	62	656	C	65
657	D	59	658	D	36	659	A	52	660	B	64
661	C	62	662	A	55	663	B	56	664	C	45
665	D	78	666	A	82	667	C	50	668	A	62
669	D	41	670	B	86	671	C	77	672	A	83
673	E	93	674	D	—	675	D	—	676	D	—
677	D	—	678	C	—	679	C	—	680	E	91
681	A	54	682	D	91	683	C	95	684	B	60
685	D	—	686	C	—	687	A	—	688	B	—
689	E	85	690	F	85	691	B	—	692	D	85
693	A	—	694	C	—	695	H	—	696	I	—
697	G	95	698	C	31	699	E	81	700	B	69
701	D	55	702	E	68	703	A	61	704	A	54
705	C	59	706	B	29	707	C	73	708	A	66
709	A	—	710	C	64	711	A	97	712	C	42
713	A	72	714	E	70	715	A	71	716	C	—
717	A	67	718	D	89	719	E	29	720	A	—
721	A	21	722	A	48	723	A	—	724	C	20
725	A	—	726	A	59	727	D	60	728	A	63
729	D	93	730	A	74	731	B	—	732	B	92
733	D	72	734	A	88	735	A	30	736	C	49
737	E	72	738	D	55	739	E	34	740	D	57
741	A	—	742	C	60	743	D	69	744	B	65
745	D	—	746	A	—	747	A	68	748	C	75
749	A	50	750	E	84	751	C	26	752	E	65
753	D	58	754	C	0	755	A	—			

Human antiparasitic chemotherapy

756	B	30	757	D	60	758	B	35	759	A	59
760	F	77	761	B	61	762	E	54	763	D	92
764	B	49	765	B	35	766	D	68	767	B	74
768	A	66	769	C	74	770	E	68	771	F	92
772	G	58	773	E	65	774	C	60	775	B	71
776	B	90	777	A	87	778	C	74	779	B	55
780	C	40	781	A	60	782	F	55	783	D	54
784	A	83	785	A	81	786	B	69	787	A	75
788	A	72	789	B	61	790	B	63	791	D	74
792	D	77	793	B	58	794	B	46	795	B	63
796	A	67	797	B	57	798	A	78	799	C	49
800	B	47	801	A	74	802	C	73	803	C	25
804	B	68	805	C	47	806	B	58	807	B	46
808	B	40	809	C	56	810	A	71	811	B	18
812	E	44	813	A	42	814	F	81	815	B	71
816	B	71	817	A	74	818	D	65	819	C	79
820	C	76	821	D	80	822	D	86	823	C	83
824	D	70	825	A	80	826	D	75	827	F	80
828	A	73	829	G	74	830	C	8	831	D	19
832	E	29	833	C	25	834	F	51	835	F	83
836	A	71	837	E	34	838	D	79	839	D	58
840	B	54	841	C	57	842	A	40	843	A	91
844	D	70	845	A	93	846	F	56	847	H	49
848	D	39	849	A	75	850	C	59	851	G	35
852	G	64	853	C	69	854	G	58	855	H	70
856	H	90	857	C	61	858	F	49	859	C	93
860	B	79	861	D	64	862	H	74	863	H	72
864	B	72	865	D	61	866	B	56	867	E	44
868	B	77	869	B	78	870	E	48	871	B	78
872	D	54	873	C	17	874	D	19	875	A	38
876	C	67	877	A	81	878	D	34	879	A	57
880	B	67	881	C	25	882	D	63	883	D	82
884	C	78	885	A	48	886	D	60	887	A	49
888	D	55	889	A	19	890	E	65			

Drug disposition and metabolism

891	A	80	892	B	—	893	C	89	894	A	85
895	B	51	896	C	64	897	D	81	898	A	46
899	C	74	900	C	94	901	B	89	902	B	86
903	D	35	904	A	41	905	C	82	906	C	71
907	A	90	908	A	79	909	B	92	910	A	88

911 B	–	912 A	15	913 A	90	914 C	72
915 B	80	916 C	95	917 C	94	918 D	78
919 E	23	920 B	80	921 C	–	922 B	74
923 C	86	924 G	–	925 C	60	926 E	54
927 C	–	928 G	–	929 A	–	930 A	89
931 C	42	932 E	87	933 H	12	934 C	63
935 E	38	936 B	58	937 G	–	938 E	88
939 D	63	940 H	49	941 E	71	942 D	56
943 E	70	944 C	29	945 F	65	946 E	18
947 B	55	948 E	–	949 C	57	950 C	–
951 B	86	952 E	–	953 E	38	954 D	15
955 E	–	956 B	70	957 C	–	958 E	–
959 B	–	960 C	–	961 B	52	962 B	83
963 C	40	964 A	–	965 A	53	966 D	65
967 E	77	968 D	–	969 E	49	970 E	70
971 A	90	972 E	55	973 A	–	974 D	29
975 C	47	976 C	–	977 A	–	978 C	–
979 A	–	980 D	15	981 A	–	982 E	–
983 C	–	984 A	–	985 D	–	986 D	–
987 C	59	988 B	74	989 C	–	990 D	–
991 D	–	992 A	–	993 E	45	994 A	–
995 D	–	996 A	–	997 E	54	998 A	49
999 E	27	1000 C	70	1001 B	68	1002 A	65
1003 G	18	1004 A	33	1005 A	55	1006 E	85
1007 D	67	1008 B	64	1009 C	72	1010 C	25
1011 B	75	1012 A	54	1013 A	43	1014 B	35
1015 C	45	1016 A	87	1017 C	20	1018 B	51
1019 A	64	1020 B	89	1021 C	79	1022 D	68
1023 F	–	1024 E	9	1025 C	53	1026 A	35
1027 C	–	1028 B	–	1029 C	37	1030 C	24
1031 D	26	1032 C	45	1033 B	26	1034 B	86
1035 B	73	1036 E	78	1037 C	94	1038 A	88
1039 A	86	1040 D	83	1041 D	92	1042 C	89
1043 A	73	1044 C	22	1045 A	38	1046 D	55
1047 E	59	1048 C	94	1049 C	56	1050 C	81
1051 A	70	1052 D	53	1053 A	96	1054 C	86
1055 E	94	1056 B	86	1057 A	94	1058 B	88
1059 B	77	1060 B	91	1061 B	59	1062 C	12
1063 C	9	1064 D	74	1065 C	78		

Applied pharmacology

1066 D	34	1067 D	85	1068 B	62	1069 B	47
1070 A	67	1071 C	78	1072 B	78	1073 C	37

1074 B	58	1075 A	–	1076 B	60	1077 B	45
1078 B	32	1079 A	44	1080 B	44	1081 D	78
1082 B	82	1083 B	78	1084 C	82	1085 C	73
1086 G	84	1087 E	26	1088 B	46	1089 A	43
1090 F	34	1091 D	17	1092 D	73	1093 E	48
1094 E	40	1095 A	95	1096 C	54	1097 F	92
1098 D	58	1099 D	56	1100 D	37	1101 A	55
1102 B	70	1103 D	60	1104 B	74	1105 E	69
1106 C	52	1107 B	69	1108 D	50	1109 A	91
1110 D	7	1111 D	86	1112 E	48	1113 G	51
1114 B	76	1115 H	93	1116 A	51	1117 A	45
1118 A	56	1119 A	51	1120 E	60	1121 C	36
1122 D	63	1123 F	54	1124 A	33	1125 A	38
1126 A	53	1127 E	73	1128 C	64	1129 B	63
1130 D	25	1131 A	74	1132 A	56	1133 E	59
1134 B	74	1135 C	92	1136 G	79	1137 F	46
1138 D	67	1139 B	89	1140 A	45	1141 E	24
1142 A	66	1143 C	81	1144 B	63	1145 E	71
1146 B	–	1147 D	–	1148 A	–	1149 C	–
1150 D	41	1151 C	59	1152 B	86	1153 A	85
1154 D	69	1155 A	21	1156 D	77	1157 B	98
1158 C	81	1159 A	74	1160 C	66	1161 A	67
1162 B	67	1163 D	46	1164 D	23	1165 D	30
1166 A	98	1167 D	77	1168 C	60	1169 C	97
1170 C	73	1171 C	95	1172 A	60	1173 E	–
1174 C	44	1175 C	43	1176 A	63	1177 C	24
1178 A	29	1179 D	26	1180 B	28	1181 A	33
1182 C	47	1183 D	53	1184 E	37	1185 E	53
1186 B	24	1187 C	57	1188 B	46	1189 B	49
1190 B	41	1191 C	43	1192 B	29	1193 B	73
1194 B	78	1195 B	–	1196 A	40	1197 A	55
1198 B	73	1199 A	60	1200 C	65